D0078174

HEALTH AND HEALING AFTER TRAUMATIC BRAIN INJURY

**Recent Title in
Disability Insights and Issues**

Surviving Cancer as a Family and Helping
Co-Survivors Thrive

Catherine A. Marshall, editor

HEALTH AND HEALING AFTER TRAUMATIC BRAIN INJURY

UNDERSTANDING THE POWER OF FAMILY, FRIENDS, COMMUNITY, AND OTHER SUPPORT SYSTEMS

Heidi Muenchberger, Elizabeth Kendall, and John Wright

Editors

Foreword by
James S. Brady,
Former White House Press Secretary

Disability Insights and Issues
Catherine A. Marshall and Elizabeth Kendall, Series Editors

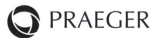 PRAEGER

AN IMPRINT OF ABC-CLIO, LLC
Santa Barbara, California • Denver, Colorado • Oxford, England

Property of
Baker College
of Allen Park

Copyright 2013 by Heidi Muenchberger, Elizabeth Kendall, and John Wright

All rights reserved. No part of this publication may be reproduced, stored in a retrieval system, or transmitted, in any form or by any means, electronic, mechanical, photocopying, recording, or otherwise, except for the inclusion of brief quotations in a review, without prior permission in writing from the publisher.

Library of Congress Cataloging-in-Publication Data

Health and healing after traumatic brain injury : understanding the power of family, friends, community, and other support systems / Heidi Muenchberger, Elizabeth Kendall, and John Wright, editors ; foreword by James S. Brady.

    p. ; cm. — (Disability insights and issues)
    Includes bibliographical references and index.
    ISBN 978-1-4408-2886-7 (hardcopy : alk. paper) — ISBN 978-1-4408-2887-4 (ebook) I. Muenchberger, Heidi. II. Kendall, Elizabeth, 1963–
    III. Wright, John, active 2012. IV. Series: Disability insights and issues.
    [DNLM: 1. Brain Injuries—rehabilitation. 2. Social Support. WL 354]
    LC Classification not assigned
    362.1974′81 — dc23   2012050993

ISBN: 978-1-4408-2886-7
EISBN: 978-1-4408-2887-4

17   16   15   14   13   1 2 3 4 5

This book is also available on the World Wide Web as an eBook.
Visit www.abc-clio.com for details.

Praeger
An Imprint of ABC-CLIO, LLC

ABC-CLIO, LLC
130 Cremona Drive, P.O. Box 1911
Santa Barbara, California 93116-1911

This book is printed on acid-free paper ∞

Manufactured in the United States of America

CONTENTS

SERIES FOREWORD

Disability is often viewed as a negative event, but what about those who thrive and flourish despite their disability? This new series is based on stories of people with disabilities and their families coping and, indeed, thriving. Readers will learn from these stories, as well as from professionals and researchers, about how best to live with and manage their disability—how to use resources in the environment, how to find peer support, and how to be in control of their treatment and service options. The series will explore the role of personal, social, and environmental supports in the process of adjusting to and managing life with a disability.

How can interventions focus on coping and thriving, rather than problems and deficits? This series will explore, for instance, what we know about strengths-based interventions, consumer-driven approaches to service delivery, and the role of creativity in coping. Juxtaposing the personal views of people with disabilities, academic evidence, and practice knowledge, we show how people with disabilities participate fully in their own lives and how they and their family members can be supported in ways that assist them in building and using resources for a positive future.

This series of authored and edited books will give readers insight into the challenges, rewards, dilemmas, and solutions facing millions of people with disabilities—disabilities developed prior to or during birth, from accident or illness, and, significant now for our population, those associated with the aging process. Disabilities addressed will include, for instance, substantial hearing or visual impairment, osteoporosis, and paralysis, as well as HIV infection, AIDS, cancer, specific learning disabilities, autism, and mobility impairments. "Hidden" disabilities such as mental illness, brain injury, chronic pain, and chronic fatigue, all of which can cause considerable misunderstanding and suffering, will also be addressed.

Series Editors
Catherine A. Marshall
Elizabeth Kendall

FOREWORD

It has now been over 30 years since my life changed permanently. It was 2:25 p.m. on a gray afternoon in March 1981, and I was standing beside former president Ronald Reagan as we left the hotel in Washington, DC. Suddenly six shots rang out across the crowd and people close to me fell to the ground. Apparently, a bullet tore through the left front of my brain. I say, apparently, because I have no memory of the event, but I have a vivid memory of the impact it has had on my life and my family.

When I reflect on it, 30 years doesn't seem so long ago really. It seems like just yesterday, but I have spent many of those years working hard with my family to regain some sense of life as I knew it. I have now spent nearly as much of my life with my brain injury as I did without it. It is difficult to think clearly about who I was at that time and who I am now as the two have blurred inextricably over the years.

What I do know clearly is that without the support and systems around me over the last 30 years, I would not be who I am today. The focus of this book is on the systems of support that can heal following brain injury. The medical and rehabilitation staff, community members who wrote countless get well cards, my former work colleagues and, most importantly, my family and friends—all these people were critical in my recovery and continue to be critical in my ongoing pursuit to create meaning from the devastation.

One of the most important resources during the last 30 years has been my own self. From the beginning, I took a positive approach to my recovery. I searched for humor wherever I could and tried to keep looking forward. My wife and I have tried to remain enthusiastic and avoid bitterness, even when this seemed impossible. I have always set myself goals and thrown myself into activities that would keep my brain active.

I have campaigned tirelessly for rehabilitation services and gun control, capitalizing on my connections and knowledge of the political and legal systems. I am proud to say that my efforts have contributed to the fact that gun laws are slowly changing in America. The Brady Bill has made a measurable impact on suicide and homicide rates, but I am deeply saddened by the recent spate of high profile gun-events similar to my own. There is still too much injury in our world caused by easy access to guns. My campaign will continue for as long as I am capable, and its impact will remain as a lasting legacy of my life. As a society, we have so much more work to do to prevent unnecessary injury and provide the type of support required by people who are struggling with this complex condition.

This book offers useful strategies to people with brain injuries, their families, health professionals and entire communities. The premise of the book is that all too often, we focus on the negatives. We prepare people for the worst, but in so doing, we can sometimes deplete them of hope and inspiration. At all levels of society, we need to have vision, passion, humanity and commitment. I still have a dream of a better society where people do not willfully hurt each other—a society where people actively seek to optimize outcomes for others, enabling people with brain injuries to flourish despite their disability. This is a laudable goal, and one to which we should all aspire. It seems so logical and achievable, but in reality, it is extremely complicated. Books like this one, that integrate the views of people with brain injuries, practitioners, policymakers and academics and focus on positive strategies, will help us move closer to this utopia. I am very proud to be associated with the book and hope it raises awareness about how we can improve the lives of those who have sustained brain injuries.

James S. Brady
Former White House Press Secretary

ACKNOWLEDGMENTS

We wish to sincerely thank the following individuals who were instrumental in the production of this publication:

Stephanie Prout and Michelle McIntyre, Editorial Assistants, Griffith University

Courtney Wright, Charmaine Jensen, Narina Jenkinson, and Dr. Annick Maujean for proofreading services

Kathryn Heinold for administrative support

Our families for their unconditional support and encouragement

The brain injury community, so wonderfully diverse and ever inspiring

PART 1

SELF-DETERMINATION AND PERSONAL HEALING AFTER TRAUMATIC BRAIN INJURY

John Wright

I didn't find out about my brain injury until exactly 20 years later. I always knew that something had changed after my accident but there was no one to talk to about this. There was certainly no rehabilitation or therapy at the time, and no one intervened when I was so obviously struggling. I just wasn't achieving the things I wanted to achieve and my life wasn't going the way I wanted it to go. No matter how hard I tried, things just didn't work out. What I now know is that this is not an uncommon story among people with brain injury. This type of experience is illustrated repeatedly in the stories contained in this section of the book. They all refer to the lack of therapy, the lack of information about brain injury, and the lack of understanding among health professionals. Irrespective of the country in which the story is based, health and rehabilitation systems have failed people with brain injuries. Perhaps systems are too rigid to ever meet the needs created by such a complex and invisible disability, but it seems to be a serious travesty of human rights that these systems can actually harm people. Those who survive the system have usually taken control themselves, seeking ways to build rehabilitation into their daily lives, finding the necessary strategies to achieve their goals and relying heavily on family and friends for support. They have persisted against sometimes insurmountable barriers and have capitalized on their strengths to accommodate their weaknesses. Like a rollercoaster ride of oscillating enthusiasm and despair, they have had to fight to overcome the compelling desire to just give up.

Often the world sends relentless messages to give up, sometimes even from those who matter most to us. Until recently, rehabilitation professionals and doctors reinforced the idea that our recovery would plateau after a few years and that we should not expect too much after that time. My own mother was told to leave me at the hospital because I would never recover. In the intervening 20 years, I have heard countless stories of similar messages, most containing derogatory terms such as vegetable. It is almost impossible to believe that such terms are used in reference to human beings. Thankfully, however, the concept of neuroplasticity has revolutionized thinking in this area, giving us hope and confirming what we already knew: that we could make things work if we kept trying and if we were given the right structures and supports. People use many terms to refer to my condition—brain injury, traumatic brain injury, acquired brain injury, head injury, head trauma. Although technically these terms may have slightly different meanings, they are used interchangeably. Irrespective of what term is used, the impact is similar.

Over the years, I have visited counselors, therapists, doctors, psychiatrists, and none have professed to know anything about brain injury. There is only a small group of professionals who have experience in this area, and this is not good enough. The stories in this book provide evidence of poorly designed rehabilitation that does not suit the needs of the individuals and their goals. They tell of wasted time spent completing tasks that did not help them to progress, of being ill-informed or poorly advised and of being misunderstood and neglected.

Most people who contributed to this section of the book highlighted the importance of family and friends, particularly when the rehabilitation system fails. Families, friends, and therapists all need to demonstrate extreme patience and tolerance when dealing with people who have brain injury. I was so fortunate to be part of a very close knit group of school friends, many of whom I still see regularly 45 years on. They helped me in profound ways during my recovery, simply by being patient, supportive, and understanding. They accommodated my problems and helped me to find new ways of doing things. They never made fun of me and they encouraged me to try everything.

However, the unpredictability of brain injury confused my friends and family. Sometimes, I could do things easily and sometimes nothing worked. To this day, if I am tired or stressed, things don't seem to go right. How is it possible for people to understand such a confusing and obscure condition? And yet, without their understanding and patience, where would we be?

If there is one thing I have learned through this process, it is never to give up. I had to be determined and tireless in my efforts to overcome the difficulties created by my injury. My mother had to be equally tireless and determined. I would have to spend many more hours than my friends or siblings if I wanted to achieve the same results. I recall walking up and down our home verandah for hours with my physiotherapist mother pushing me along. I owe my physical recovery to her determination, but I still exercise every day to prevent my paralysis from taking over the right side of my body, stiffening my muscles and contracting my limbs. The people who contributed to this section of the book all describe similar effort and persistence. They describe the need to take, and be given, sufficient time to rebuild their strength and ability at their own pace. They have all reached for big ambitions and, even if they haven't quite made it, they have progressed well beyond what was expected for them.

However, it is difficult to maintain the necessary level of determination in the face of the devastating changes and losses created by brain injury. After my accident, I changed from being a talented young person to one who struggled with daily tasks. From top of my class scholastically, my grades plummeted and I lost confidence—I could no longer keep up at school. I had always been sought after on every sporting team because I could do anything, but after my accident, I couldn't even walk properly. I was so uncoordinated that I constantly dropped the ball and came last in every race. These physical problems impacted on my confidence even further. Prior to my accident, I was one of the most social kids in school and was known for my ability to mix with a wide range of friends of all ages. I was famous for my funny once-at-home . . . stories through which I entertained my friends for hours.

After my accident, a stranger lived in my body—he was inappropriate, disinhibited, verbose, and aggressive. I felt as if I was no longer in control of my own actions or thoughts. In the subsequent years, this new personality lost me many friendships and burned many bridges that I have regretted deeply. The stories in this section of the book similarly talk about the contrast between their views of themselves and their postinjury abilities. They describe how long it took to come to terms with the massive changes associated with their injuries and how difficult it was to understand the differences. They also describe the disproportionate impact of subtle changes that were even more difficult to understand and almost impossible to explain to anyone else.

Over the years, through hard work and persistence, I have managed to tame my new personality a little. I have certainly recovered physically from my injury. Although I still have some residual weakness, I am now fitter and more active than most men my age, but this has taken enormous determination and effort. I made it through college and eventually learned to control my brain when it threatened to take me on an irrelevant journey. I am sure some people still wonder why I am a bit different, but I have capitalized on the notion of being eccentric and have learned to use it to my advantage. My disinhibition, which was so destructive in the early days, now allows me to engage with new people and exciting places or gain information that would not be accessible to those who are more reserved. People eventually learn to accept me this way and some have even followed suit or benefited from my openness. My greatest pleasure came when my grown up daughter commented about how lucky I was to be so at ease with myself. In comparison to how constrained most people are in society, she noticed how free I was to express myself fully.

Yes, I can certainly see the silver lining in my brain injury. I have had to do so in order to survive as have most of the people who have contributed to this section of the book. They all talk about opportunities that would not have emerged without having experienced brain injury. They describe the importance of remaining positive, having fun, and re-evaluating life to deemphasize the losses. Many of them refer to their injury as a new start at life, grateful for having survived, but indelibly changed by the experience. In some ways, brain injury is like a process of being reborn, but as a slightly different person. In my case, my injury has allowed me to relate better to people, to understand hardship and not be dismissive about others' distress. It has given me compassion and a sense of humanity that allows me to help others and contribute to society in meaningful ways. However, I will never recover from the deep sadness that engulfs me every time I think about what might have been had I not been injured. No silver lining can ever remove this sadness—intense sadness and happiness always coexist in a poignant and perpetual emotional interaction. We must establish systems of support that can help each person who sustains a brain injury to manage this sadness but still reach for the potential that neuroplasticity can offer. This potential will be maximized when those with brain injuries can embrace self-determination and still draw on supportive families, helpful accepting communities, and skillful health professionals.

FREEDOM

Sky above gravity: where clouds go, stars float, the sun baths, and
    moon sways
Waiting for a chance to never look back asking, *is this all right?*
A smile carved of everything right.
No more hesitation of presentation of all things questionable
What is free?
There. That's it! Can't you see? A girl riding a noble steed.
A girl on a horse embodies all things free.
Gliding over earthly woes.
Nothing but the sky when looking up
Four legs open the gate to freedoms wild place, tasting the winds of
    melting chains
A girl on a horse is nothing more than freedom welcoming one more
A girl who needs so many things can give them all away on a day
    where flying out of a cage comes with a wild mane.
What is free?
There. That's it! Can't you see? It's not such a big mystery.
A girl on a noble steed is freedom ringing clearly.

Erica Anderson

CHAPTER 1

Advice From the Heart: Stories of Survival and Growth Following Brain Injury

Lisa Guttentag Lederer

I am Lisa Guttentag. My accident happened on June 12, 2000. I had just completed my first year at Harvard University in Boston, and my joyful memories of close friendships formed during that year, along with the thrill of having the opportunity to attend such a renowned place, made me foolishly feel invincible. As I drove my family's minivan on a busy street in Greensboro, North Carolina, with the mundane aim of buying a bathing suit—though I do not remember the morning—I must have been less focused on the road than usual. I was thinking about my internship at a biological research station in Australia, which was to begin in three days. Apparently, I failed to notice a tractor-trailer ploughing toward me as I made a left turn.

I was kept in an induced coma for three days and remained in a coma for 13 days after the drugs were stopped. Doctors first predicted that I would die; then, after I had remained alive for several days, that I would live in a permanent vegetative state; and then, after I emerged from the coma that I would leave the hospital in three months for a group home. My prognosis kept improving. As my second month in the hospital began, my life became an all-enveloping endeavor to defy more of the doctors' predictions.

On the rehabilitation ward, I would begin each morning by carefully memorizing the therapy schedule posted daily on my bathroom door—a slip of paper with numerous time slots filled with "physical," "occupational," "speech," and "recreational." For me, that schedule had become a new life story each day. Therapy was my future. What I knew of the past of the girl named Lisa Guttentag, though I worked desperately to continue the story of her life, was a distant beacon that some magical recipe of daily therapies would allow me to reach. I toiled at therapy, relearning to talk and walk, with the childlike determination of a person focused entirely on a single goal. Now I suspect that, with the aim of becoming the former Lisa planted firmly in my head, I had no room in my rattled brain for anything else. Whatever the reason, I spent every waking hour working to "get better"—to become Lisa Guttentag again.

After two months in the hospital, I was finally allowed to go home; but my focus on finding a magical recipe of therapeutic daily activities continued. For the first eight weeks, I attended outpatient therapy three times a week. My therapists at the hospital had been eager to devise creative strategies to help me progress, but those at outpatient seemed to run mechanically through the same formula of therapy with me and every head-injured person. I felt that my own specific deficits, instead of being treated, were squeezed into a special mold so that they could fit in the tick boxes on assessment forms. I remember sitting on the edge of the plastic mats used for physical therapy exercises, lonely and frustrated but resigned, surrounded by people dutifully carrying out standardized routines.

My head injury resulted in several physical deficits, but it did not cause short-term memory loss or impulsiveness, as do many. For me, the more important effects revolved around my emotions: I had none. The complacency I felt on those plastic mats at therapy, in fact, is almost all I have felt for the last two years.

When I sat on those mats, I would realize with a sort of mental dread that, before my accident, my stomach would have been fluttering, or heaving, or at least tightening with frustration or sorrow. But the appropriate bodily responses to my imagined emotions no longer occurred. I never cried, because I never felt sad; when I laughed, it was because I knew I ought to laugh, and it had all the sickening blankness of a fake chuckle. I often repeated to myself, "I am sad, I am sad, I am sad," or, "I am happy, I am happy, I am happy;" but I never had the triumphant feeling that I had overcome any sadness, or tamed any happiness, in order to pursue my goals. Instead, my imagined emotions continued to swirl disturbingly in my mind. I stared at the world, as I think my relatives and friends detected, with an uncaring "deadness." The few people I told about the deadness, however, seemed reluctant to believe me, and even if they did, they found it difficult to comprehend why an inability to feel sadness would disturb anyone.

The obvious physical effects of my injury—which include a loss of coordination in my right hand, reduced sensation throughout my left side, difficulty pronouncing words, and double vision in my lower visual field—have naturally disrupted my daily activities. Much more disrupting, however, have been the cognitive and emotional changes that have occurred over time. I can describe one of my states of mind as deadness because I can contrast it with the "aliveness" that has slowly crept back into my body. Now, I have regained the ability to cry, though only briefly from my right eye. Although it is difficult to pinpoint how exactly it has changed, my perception of the world has continuously changed so radically during the past two years that I feel that I am now operating on an entirely different cognitive system than I was even a few months ago.

I have since mechanically churned my way through Harvard and have even spent a summer at the biological research station in Australia, for which I was headed when I crashed my van. Much more significant, though, was the summer I spent as an intern for the Waikato Head Injury Society of New Zealand. Here, I had the opportunity to interview a score of people with brain injuries, recording the following stories that simply demanded to be written. The stories were eagerly shared in the hope that they would help others with head injury in the future. I emerged from my adventures in New Zealand frustrated and, at times, socially isolated, but hopeful—not only mentally hopeful, but the kind of hopeful that makes my heart beat faster. Although I am ecstatic to be recovering some of my emotion, I am angered that so few medical professionals recognize head injury or have an understanding of the bizarreness of its effects.

This chapter is a compilation of the stories I was told in New Zealand. From them, I have learned that no one with a head injury has a standard set of deficits, nor is there some magical formula through which people with head injuries become their former selves. We all find our own way, first of managing to wait for physiological changes that can be the building blocks of a life—part reinvigorated and part new—and then, of thriving.

Brett's Story

"There is life after head injury," promises Brett. But he has expressed this belief far more through his actions than through his words.

When Brett was training for a bicycle race on December 12, 1990, he did not suspect that it would be necessary to ponder head injury. He had taken up long-distance cycling the previous year because, he says, "I really enjoyed pushing myself to the max." Between Cambridge and Te Awamutu, Brett was going over 40 kmph when the rider in front of him fell off his bicycle. Brett was sent hurtling over the crashed bicycle onto the road, and only his helmet saved his life. The race he had been training for, the Whangamata race of 125 kilometers, did not even take place that year.

Brett remained in a coma for two days and in the hospital for seven days in all. During that time though, doctors treated his relatively minor physical injuries. No one discussed head injury with him. "I thought there was nothing wrong with me," he recounts. "I walked okay, I talked okay, and

I looked normal. As far as I could tell, nothing was the matter." He was so convinced of this that he managed to escape from the hospital, apparently sneaking out in everyday clothes and trekking several kilometers to his house. "I was lucky I wasn't run over," he admits. When he could not find his wife at home, he visited his neighbors, who politely gave him a cup of tea and then wisely phoned the hospital to inform them of where to find their missing patient, "that says something about my determination," reflects Brett, "and it also says I knew nothing about head injury."

When he was officially released from the hospital, Brett was still oblivious to the deficits his head injury had caused, "no one told me, 'Brett, you've changed; Brett, you shouldn't be doing that.' And I'm still quite angry about that," he asserts. He says that if someone had informed him of his own mental problems, he would have been spared a good deal of pain and frustration, "I kept trying and failing, trying and failing," he reports, "my life turned to custard."

After leaving the hospital, Brett quickly resumed his job teaching at an Intermediate School. However, he observes that at that point, "teaching was no longer a job for me." Brett would lose track of what he had planned to do in each lesson and of the progress each student had made. He often forgot the students' names. Lacking his former patience, he began, as he says, "lashing out at kids giving me grief." Dealing with thirty kids at once quickly overwhelmed him. "I lost my ability to multitask," he explains. Finally, in 1993, he had to resign.

As Brett realized, the life he had painstakingly carved out for himself before his accident was quickly dissolving. He says emphatically, "I had worked hard to get where I was in life, and I thought I'd be there for the rest of my life." His degree and teaching diploma, earned through five years at university, had become useless to him. Yet the most significant losses for him were less tangible parts of his life. "After a serious head injury," he asserts, "you lose your old self, your relationships . . . and usually your career." Brett landed in court and nearly in jail. At the same time, because he had no visible disabilities, it was difficult for people to accept that he had any disabilities at all. "I wish," he muses, "as the result of my accident, I chopped an arm or a leg off so I could hold up a stump and say, 'Look here, I'm disabled.' " In 1993, when Brett's first daughter was born, he came close to committing suicide.

With the birth of his daughter, however, Brett's life began to change. He now has two daughters, aged nine and four, and he says earnestly, "they've given me something to live for." After he lost his teaching job, Brett finally learned from a psychiatrist who researched his hospital records that he had sustained a serious head injury. The psychiatrist referred him to the Waikato Head Injury Society. Brett had become socially withdrawn after his accident, but he quickly met friends through the Head Injury Society and became involved in its management, serving as the editor of the newsletter and recently as the president. Throughout the past nine years, Brett has worked tirelessly to prevent other head-injured people from facing the same frustration that nearly destroyed him. He has proved that his habit of pushing himself "to the max" did not end with his injury. With the help of the diary he now carries everywhere, Brett has reorganized his life and has become an enthusiastic spokesperson for the head-injured, "to coin a phrase," he smiles, "I'm a bit stuffed in the head . . . but that doesn't stop me!"

After he left teaching, Brett devoted his energy to building up a vintage car collection, which soon became his own business, Hudson Hire. Besides helping people through some of the toughest times of their lives at the Head Injury Society, he adds balance to his life by running Hudson Hire, driving people to and from one of the happiest events in their lives: their wedding. "Far less stress and grief in doing that as a job, than teaching," he smiles.

Brett's advice to other head-injured people is so polished, and it is evident he has pondered it for a long time. He scribbles down some notes, as he often does, to organize his thoughts, and then announces authoritatively, "It is unlikely that life is ever going to be the same. There are going to be changes. But some of those changes are good, not bad. Look at me. Since my injury, I've started my own business. I have two wonderful girls, and my wife and I have remained together. I've become a Christian, which has meant more to me than earning my teaching degree through five years of work. I've run a marathon. And I've done the Whangamata bike ride for which I was training when I had my accident—three times, the last time in less than four hours!" Glancing around the office of the Head Injury Society, Brett adds, "I now have a real understanding and empathy for those who are less fortunate, for those who have had major trauma in life."

Derek's Story

"Non legitae carborundum," Derek carefully pronounces each word. He smiles. "It's my favorite Latin expression. It means, 'Don't let them grind you down.' "

Derek's battle against being ground down began 12 years ago, when he had been working as an English teacher in Japan for six months. He remembers waiting at his friend's apartment to go to a party. "The next thing I know, I was waking up in Auckland Hospital, which is in a different country, and it was some months later." He was told that he had fallen off the top of a six-story building.

Derek learned at Auckland Hospital that he had been in a coma for five-and-a-half months. Upon his arrival at the hospital, the doctor had given him a 0 percent chance of survival. "After a week," he recounts, "I still hadn't died, so they put it up to a 10 percent chance of survival." He grins, and then corrects himself, "I actually did die, a couple of times. But they started me up again."

When Derek returned to Japan five years later, the doctor who had cared for him after the accident performed a magnetic resonance imaging (MRI) scan of his brain. It was then that Derek learned more about what had happened inside his head. He recalls, "I could see slice-by-slice exactly what was wrong with it. Even five years after the accident, there was still a big, dark blotch in the frontal lobes."

The effects of that big, dark blotch have dominated Derek's life ever since. He spent a year in total at Auckland and Middlemore Hospitals and then went home to live with his mother. He recalls only brief segments of his time at home because he was "only vaguely aware of what was happening" at the time. Ever since the accident 12 years ago, he explains, "You could say that I was slowly recovering." It seems to Derek that the process of his "waking up," or climbing through states of consciousness, has continued for the past 12 years.

Derek remembers being semilucid for the first few years after leaving the hospital. "That was one word I learned after waking up," he remembers. At the hospital, he explains, "I found I really expanded my vocabulary, because the only thing I could do for a long time . . . was crosswords."

Though he had never done crossword puzzles before his accident, Derek struggles through them in the hospital as a way of passing time, learning how to write again, and as he says, exercising his "powers of recollection." Although the physical therapy he attended four days a week seemed beneficial, he was not challenged by the occupational and cognitive therapy that he received at the hospital. He complains, "It was just really, really basic stuff." Derek quickly adds, "mind you, I suppose it was for the severely impaired. I just found that I quickly recovered beyond what they could help me with. But OT [occupational therapy] was better than doing nothing. And I used to spend far too much time doing nothing in hospital." The television programs that captured the attention of most patients on the ward—"soap operas and that," as Derek describes them—bored him. Crossword puzzles became the primary element of his rehabilitation and a central focus of his life. Initially, he says, "It was very hard . . . for a long time, I couldn't finish any of them. After a while, I sort of managed to finish them; first of all, it was a cause of celebration." The memory makes him smile, "and it's a habit that stuck; I still really love crosswords."

Derek went from hospital to his mother's house, where he lived for two years until she was diagnosed with a brain tumor. After her death, he lived in Auckland for a year at a physical rehabilitation center, where the therapy, happily, proved more beneficial than that at the hospital.

Derek admits that he has some challenging deficits from his head injury. He says he continues to have memory problems and has difficulty thinking logically. His left side is still weak, and he can only leave his wheelchair to walk with a stick. Many of his friendships, both those that began before the accident and those that began afterward, have suffered.

Derek reports that, "generally, a lot of people don't know how to treat me, so they just don't treat me."

Yet despite these problems, Derek is actually pleased about some of his cognitive and emotional disabilities, which he says have forced him into a more methodical approach to problem-solving. "I think I'm much more analytical now . . . I've had to be. It's more of an adaptive thing." Later, he explains, "I'm more able to focus on one thing at a time. I had to discipline myself to focus on one thing more intently, because otherwise I couldn't achieve even a simple goal." He feels less driven by emotion and more content overall, "Emotionally, I've been much better than I was before my accident." He smiles. "I was a pretty grim character back then." In his everyday life, perhaps because he is not as grim, Derek has also become more eager to interact with other people. His new friendliness, he says, "seemed to be reciprocal . . . sometimes it's good, because I get a bit tired, and someone offers me a push. I appreciate it."

It is not surprising that people offer to push Derek's wheelchair. He is always inventively finding a way, even if it is difficult, to do what he wants to do. Every morning, he propels himself about five kilometers to a local cafe for morning tea. He comments that he has always been a creative person. Before he taught English in Japan, he was studying at a creative arts school in the hope of finding a job that would allow him to use his creativity. "I try to 'think outside the square,' " Derek says, "and I've sort of taken that and applied it to life. So now I . . . live outside the square, as well. I just treat problem-solving on a case-by-case basis, not relying on any . . . pre-held beliefs, or anything like that." He reflects, "I find that makes life more fun too, because it makes every experience like a new experience." He smiles. "I think that's how life should be."

Helen's Story

After 3 hours and 45 minutes, Helen crossed the finish line. Helen had walked five kilometers with her walker in front of her, her caregivers, family, and friends on either side. This was the second time she had walked in the Hamilton Marathon. In last year's race, her mother had pushed her in the wheelchair she usually uses. That time, when Helen completed the race, she had announced that, the next year, she wanted to walk with only her walking frame to support her.

Of course, Helen did not use words to make this announcement. She used the special language she and her caregiver have devised. Helen spells out most words letter by letter, using sounds for some and gestures to represent those that are especially difficult for her to pronounce. For the letter "I" she blinks her eyes; for "U" she looks upwards. She also uses signs for some words: a hand to her ear for "phone" and clicking noises for "horseback riding."

Helen is 31 years old. She had been a machinist for eight years when, on March 19, 1994, her car was hit near her home by another car that came around a curve on the wrong side. As usual, she had been waiting to reach the main road before fastening her seat belt. When doctors performed a computed tomography (CT) scan to check for brain injury, Helen went into cardiac arrest, and the oxygen supply to her brain was cut off. When she was resuscitated, no one was sure how extensive the damage to her brain would be. Doctors initially warned Helen's parents to prepare for the worst. It wasn't until last year that her parents learned from a neurologist exactly where and how her brain had been damaged. Helen's mother reports that, "he was looking at the file. It was on file, but nobody had ever told us. They gave us little bits of information along the way, but not what we wanted to hear."

Helen stayed in the hospital for seven months. She attended physical and occupational therapy three times a week, gradually preparing to re-enter the world. When she came home, she was in a wheelchair and had only limited use of one arm and hand. Helen's right hand—her "ugly hand" as she calls it—is paralyzed, with the fingers curled. Most importantly to her, she is blind and cannot speak.

During her first few months at home, Helen wanted to die, "she wanted us to help her do it," says her mother. "We told her we had come too far at that stage; get up and do it yourself if you're going to do it." Sharron, Helen's caregiver, has looked after her for seven years. She turns toward Helen, "you asked me on numerous occasions to do it for you as well. Didn't you?" she recalls, "if Helen was capable of doing it, she would have killed herself. But it was a physical impossibility for Helen to get up and do it."

Sharron reports that there was a good deal of head-banging during those first months. Helen smiles sheepishly. That was a period, she says, when Helen wanted desperately to associate with normal friends instead of with handicapped people. "I told her that other handicapped people felt normal inside their heads too," she points out.

As Helen slowly accepted her disabilities, her family also had to become used to the new Helen who could not walk, see, or speak. I ask whether this new Helen is different, not just externally, but personally, "well," her mother pauses, "not a great deal, no. She still likes dirty jokes . . . and loud music." All three laugh. Although she feels her personality remained the same after the accident, many of Helen's closest normal friends lost touch for a while, and have now, as Sharron says, "gone on their merry way." She says to Helen, "you still have a bit of a problem with that. Helen feels she hasn't changed inside, and it's been hard to make new friends because of your speech . . . When we would go to functions at the Blind Foundation, because these people were blind, we would have to explain that, yes, Helen has a lot of disabilities; and yes, Helen can't speak; but yes, Helen can understand. We've got to go through all that rigmarole all the time, so that's probably frustrating and horrible for Helen to hear that all the time, for us to go around saying to people . . ." Helen interrupts, voicing some words that only Sharron is practiced enough to understand. Sharron translates, "I've put up with it. I'm over it."

During the past two years, Helen has taken the first two airplane trips in her life, to Brisbane and Sydney with Sharron. The airline staff on her first flight were not prepared to serve a disabled person, hoisting her over the armrests to the window seat for safety reasons and banging her head on the ceiling. However, both she and Sharron say that first trip changed Helen's outlook on life, "I learned I had a life," Helen says emphatically.

Helen will attend physical, occupational, and speech therapy regularly for the rest of her life. After my interview, she was going to hospital with Sharron for physiotherapy on her right hand. She has improved her dexterity by attending a craft group with Sharron, and for several years has improved her balance and muscle tone, besides gaining a love for riding horses, at Riding for the Disabled.

Helen and her family realize that they will someday face the challenge of finding housing for her. She knows the day will come when her parents can no longer care for her; Helen says she worries about finding reliable caregivers. If a caretaker fails to arrive at her home one morning, she cannot even lift herself out of bed. However, this worry is overshadowed by Helen's dread of entering a nursing home, "we don't talk much about that part of the future," admits her mother, "It's too scary."

Although, eventually they will have more difficulties to face, Helen and her family have achieved so far what was believed to be impossible. To families and friends of head-injured people, Sharron urges, "your focus is initially on what's going on, on a day-to-day basis. For everybody, for the brain injury survivor and for their families, at some stage they need to shift that focus to the future . . . and think, well, yes, that person does have a life, and it may not be the life anybody had envisaged. But if you can look beyond that, look toward the future and think, there are aims, and dreams, and goals. That, I think, is probably what brings every person through." She pauses, "and in relation to help, just asking the agencies that are out there, you've just got to keep knocking on doors . . . you've just got to keep going harder, you can never stop. You have to keep going, and going, and going . . . those people that have been through it, they're great people to go knocking on their doors and saying, 'where do we go from here?' " Helen adds a straightforward piece of advice, "go hard."

Participants in one of Helen's 5 km walks this year were supposed to wear funny hats, "no one did, of course," laughs Sharron, "except Helen." Two years ago, the first walk was more difficult for Helen because her feet were unaccustomed to the pressure of walking; it required months of training. One of Helen's caregivers nominated her for the Blind Achiever's Award for Sport for her "determination and sheer guts." She won the opportunity to attend a banquet at the government house in Wellington with the governor general.

After that banquet, Sharron read a speech that Helen had composed, which ended with a quote, "If you can imagine it, you can achieve it. If you can dream it, you can become it."

Mark's Story

Today, Mark is an expert website designer and an avid caver. Before his head injury, he was neither of these.

In 1988, Mark had a motor vehicle accident while driving at high speed. For the three weeks he was in hospital, doctors worked only on mending his visible fractures and lacerations. The signs of a head injury were not clear until after he returned home, when his strange, sometimes belligerent behavior began to concern both Mark and his family.

He laughs, "when you're in the garden and you wallop your son for making a little mistake, you know something's wrong." Before the accident, Mark says he had been "a perfectionist; an outgoing yuppie snob." Afterward, he became a recluse. He describes how he went from confidently addressing company directors to worrying about talking to a stranger. His visible physical injuries intensified his shyness, until someone else who had been in a car accident showed Mark a photograph of his own ghastly injuries, "they had all healed," explains Mark, "and I was relieved."

Mark's insurer judged his problems, including aphasia and difficulty with language, which usually resulted from head trauma, to be preexisting. At first, Mark was assigned to receive rehabilitation from Mental Health Services, which placed him in counseling with people suffering from depression and other emotional problems. When he finally received more appropriate therapy in the form of a furniture-making course, Mark was pleased to discover that he enjoyed woodworking. At the course, he met someone who offered him a job building houses and he eagerly agreed to begin work.

Although Mark liked construction work, he admits that the job was not ideal for a head-injured person, "I would get tired," he admits, "and do stupid things. I nailed myself with a nail gun once. That hurt . . . " After a year of construction work, Mark prudently quit the job and became a contract worker on a dairy farm. There, because he fatigued easily, he would spend four or five hours working in the morning, take a three-hour nap at lunch, and then spend more time working in the afternoon. Finally, when the job became too exhausting, Mark signed on as the instructor of a computer training course for kids. This new job occupied only 20 hours a week, but the company that he worked for insisted that he fill 30. His fatigue got the better of him and he was soon forced to quit.

At that point, Mark says that he and his wife "switched roles." He became the house-husband, caring for their four-year-old son and two-year-old daughter. Isolated from the friends he was used to seeing in a work environment, Mark became lonely and depressed.

His insurer provided him with little information or support. "My rehabilitation?" Mark chuckles, "it consisted of someone coming and telling me how to use a diary again." Eventually, however, he was able to glean more information about head injury and better understand his difficulties. Because he was a perfectionist before the accident, he says, "It was really hard to learn it's okay to make mistakes." Finally someone stressed to him that, "there ain't a cure" for brain injury, so Mark accepted that mistakes were going to be made. Now more tolerant of his errors, Mark advises other people with head injury to be patient, "give it time, learn to laugh, and have fun."

Today, Mark spends much of his time updating the websites he designed for several organizations. He says the support and information from the Head Injury Society has been important to him. Mark has met several friends at the society who are eager to participate in his new hobby of caving. He soon plans to lead interested members on a trip through the Waitomo Caves. He adds to his suggestion for head-injured people to "try something completely new."

Debby's Story

After Debby's head injury, her friends left her, and she lost her prospects for a job as a medical assistant with the navy. But she says honestly, laughing, "I wasn't really concerned."

Debby remembers when she was 17 years old, in 1981, driving to a horseback riding center with friends. She later learned that the car had rolled over a bank. Debby spent "three or four months" in a coma—she is not sure exactly how long—and 18 months in the hospital. While there, she attended physiotherapy in a swimming pool once a week, but it was her mum, once a nurse, who taught her to walk and talk again after she returned home. She had no broken bones, as far as she knows, but she had lost some of her hearing ability and one eye in the accident. For a few years, although she did activities at a rehabilitation center, she says they did not benefit her much because, as she puts it simply, she was never "a crafty person."

As she watched her life fall apart, Debby laughed and built a new life. Before her accident, she had worked as an essayist. Only two months after she left hospital, she received a phone call to schedule an interview for a position as a medical assistant in the navy, as she had planned to do before her accident. Debby explains that she had been attracted by the idea of, "going around the world for nothing." However, her disabilities precluded her from taking the job. Not liking to be idle, she took a number of volunteer jobs, "I love working. I hate sitting at home . . . crying about things. I like to get out and meet people."

One year after she moved home, Debby used her compensation payment to buy her own house. Fiercely independent, she fell into her new way of life almost as quickly as her old one had ended, "mum said I was a fighter," she says, "you have to look out for yourself, and I did." Because she knew that she could no longer participate in the sports she had loved, she replaced them with other activities. She laughs, "I had to do slow stuff, like playing bowls, which I thought was an old people's game." She feels that she has changed mentally, not because of her head injury but because her physical disabilities have given her a fresh perspective. She reflects, "I think quite differently, now . . . when you're disabled, you get a different view of life." Her disabilities forced her to accept a new, often disconcerting, reaction from people when they first meet her. "People just stand there and stare at me as I walk, because my leg sticks out." Debby smiles, "people don't take me as I am, so . . .," she shrugs.

It was at one of her volunteer jobs at LIFE Unlimited, a resource center for disabled people, that Debby first met Barry in 1984. "I was all insecure inside me about meeting boys and things like that. I didn't think anyone would be interested in me," she admits. Barry and Debby had been dating for some time when his house burned down, and her mother suggested that he move in with her. Two years later, on April Fool's Day, Barry, who uses a wheelchair, "popped the question." "He actually hopped on his knee and asked me," Debby laughs. "I don't know if he actually just fell out of his chair, or if he did it on purpose." Though he initially asked her in the morning, because it was April Fool's Day, "I sort of ignored him, so he asked again in the afternoon," she shrugs. Now, the two are happily married and both still work at LIFE Unlimited.

Debby's advice for head-injured people is not surprising, coming from someone who has always "looked out for herself" and who laughs so much. "Stand on your own two feet, as much as you can," she says simply. "Be positive, don't be too negative. When you're negative, things start going downhill . . . You've got to be as positive as you can be."

Julie's Story

Less than four months before this interview, Julie was in a coma. A little over two months prior, she stopped begging to be released from hospital. She laughs, "I was just sitting there, bugging and bugging the nurses, 'can I go home? Can I go home? Can I get discharged today? Can I go home?' "

Julie is 17 years old. On March 7, 2011, she was crossing the road to get pizza after leaving her job at a factory, a job she hoped would allow her to earn enough money to afford an exciting vacation. The last thing she remembers from that afternoon is waiting in the median strip in the center of the road when she saw a car approaching. The car, going 70 kmph in a 50 kmph zone, hit Julie on the median strip. After Julie arrived at the hospital, she was put in a drug-induced coma for "four weeks and three days." Recovery after the coma came gradually. In physical and occupational therapy, Julie began to walk and talk again. At first, she was unable to read due to vision problems and was barred from watching television, which doctors feared would overstimulate her brain, "I wasn't really allowed to do anything," she says, grimacing, "I wasn't even allowed to walk down the hall by myself." Julie ponders a moment, and then smiles. She recounts, "every time the nurses would come in, they would go, 'Ah, how are you today, Julie?' And I would say, 'Bored!'"

After she was released from hospital, Julie spent six weeks in a residential rehabilitation center, where she had intensive therapy every day. Bit by bit, she relearned the routines, like cleaning her room and doing laundry that had once been an unconscious part of her everyday life. "I couldn't decide things," she explains. "It was really hard, because . . . cleaning my bedroom, I'd go, 'What do I do first?—ooh, aah, how do I do this?'"

When Julie first came home from the rehabilitation center, she was prepared to face some major obstacles. She says, "they thought it would be a really big shock mentally and physically, because I'd be doing a lot more." Ironically, the accident helped Julie and her mum "get along even better." The atmosphere inside Julie's home became more relaxed, but activities outside of it became more and more difficult for her. She had trouble recognizing some of her friends, and even as she gradually came to remember more about them, she discovered that spending time with them quickly fatigued her. She explains they are "in a party phase," so being unable to drive or spend long periods of time with other people is particularly frustrating. "If I get 'tiddly' [slightly drunk] . . . I might fall over and smack my head again," she laughs. "There's a lot of consequences I have to think about now, and my friends don't . . . I can't really keep up with them anymore." Even the friends she was once close to are now hesitant to see her. "They don't know how to talk to me anymore. They . . . look at me . . . and they're just so puzzled. In a way, it's made it really kind of lonely. It's made me feel like the old me's gone, in some ways." She pauses reflectively, "and I wonder if that's good or bad." In many ways, Julie has decided the "new" her is an improvement on the old, "before," she explains, "I was just being a silly teenager . . . partying all the time. The accident however, made me realize, slow down, think about life . . . I'm pretty much sorting out my life, for a change."

Now, although she is still getting used to the changes she has had to make since her accident, Julie has reshaped her life. Instead of pursuing a degree in travel and tourism as she had planned, she now hopes to study health science at a polytechnic. Next semester, she plans to complete correspondence courses in human biology, English, and computers as she works toward her new goal.

Julie advises other people with head injury to have the same resilience. "Don't let it get to you, because you're not dead. There's a lot you can still do," she asserts. She emphasizes the importance of finding a friend to talk to, like the boy she met and befriended in hospital. She smiles, "We were always talking . . . It was good to know someone who went through the same thing as me . . . I still go visit him."

The determination that pulled Julie through the last four months is evident in her interactions with people. After we finish talking, she notes that I am left-handed. I admit that I was actually right-handed until my own accident impaired coordination in my dominant hand. She excitedly instructs me to write my name twice with my right hand, and I painstakingly comply.

She looks at the script and says enthusiastically, "see? Look. The second time you wrote it was better than the first! Just one time is enough to make it better!" She suggests that we write letters to each other with our weak hands. It is clear that Julie is earnest when she gives this advice to head-injured people, "have a really good, positive attitude . . . just try your hardest. Life's always good, if you make it good."

CHAPTER 2

Neuroplasticity and Mindfulness in Brain Injury Rehabilitation: Cause for Great Optimism

Anita Chauvin, Michelle McIntyre, and Glyn Blackett

Research in the field of "neuroplasticity" has increasingly garnered popular attention over last decade, and brought great optimism for people with brain injuries. Studies have concluded that the brain continues to develop and remains malleable, or *plastic* throughout life (Arden, 2010; Arrowsmith-Young, 2012; Doidge, 2010). Neuroplasticity refers to the capacity for the brain to reorganize its structure, function, and neural connections in response to internal and external stimuli (Cramer et al., 2011). Recent literature describes new understandings about neuroplasticity, explaining that brain structure continues to develop throughout life in response to experiences; that the physical and cognitive abilities we are born with can be enhanced; that dead brain cells can sometimes be replaced; and that the injured brain can often reorganize itself, substituting injured parts for non-injured parts (Doidge, 2010). This literature also explains how neuroplasticity can be intentionally directed through physical and cognitive activities. Brain plasticity suggests it may be possible to rewire neural connections; activate new pathways; improve synchrony of thoughts, feelings, and emotions; improve responsiveness to and connection with others; and improve ongoing recovery and development.

Neuroplasticity involves processes of regeneration and reorganization that occur naturally in the brain throughout life, and can be evaluated at multiple levels including molecular, cellular, systemic, and behavioral adaptations (Cramer et al., 2011; Young & Tolentino, 2011). In a positive development for neuro-rehabilitation, neuroplasticity can be manipulated using a variety of approaches including neuropharmacology, brain stimulation therapies, surgical techniques, physical practices, and cognitive training (Cramer et al., 2011). Implicit in the physical and cognitive approaches to neuroplasticity is the idea that people can actively change the neural pathways in their brain. By working with specific parts of the brain, people can learn to become more calm and attentive, to improve memory skills, to reduce depression and increase feelings of well-being, and to re-gain lost function, all of which have relevance to people with traumatic brain injury (TBI). The idea that we can alter our brain gives hope that we can actively support optimal recovery after brain injury.

However, not all neuroplastic changes are positive. For instance, pain or maladaptive coping strategies can reinforce undesirable brain adaptation, leading to chronic pain or nervous system dysfunction. This underscores the need to ensure that rehabilitation programs induce desired plasticity and enhance, rather than hinder, spontaneous recovery (Kolb, Muhammad, & Gibb, 2011). Understanding how to optimize brain plasticity and direct plasticity to desired outcomes is now the focus of current research.

Discovery of Neuroplasticity and Ongoing Research

Early understanding of the brain suggested there were a fixed number of neurons, and that the brain with which you were born was the same brain with which you would die (Arden, 2010). This mechanistic notion of the brain as fixed meant that ideas of strengthening or healing the brain were not considered, allowing little hope that the brain could biologically recover from traumatic injury. However, with the use of more sophisticated technology such as functional magnetic resonance imaging (fMRI) and positron emission topography (PET) scans, it became apparent that the brain continues to develop throughout the lifetime, establishing novel neural connections, giving credence to the theory of neuroplasticity.

Prior to the insights about brain plasticity learned through the use these modern technologies, some early researchers had suggested that prevailing understandings about the "fixed" nature of the brain were incorrect. In the 1940s Polish neurophysiologist Jerzy Konorski first introduced the term neuroplasticity to describe the changes in brain function he observed when rehabilitating injured soldiers after World War II. Konorski posited that the brain was able to "modify, strengthen, and create as well as eliminate, synaptic connections" (Zielinski, 2006, cited in DeFina et al., 2009, p. 1392). This work was extended by Hebb (1949) who examined *use-induced* changes to the central nervous system. Although research conducted on animals throughout the 1950s showed that the brains of rodents changed in response to environment, it was not until 1998 that Erikkson and colleagues found evidence for plasticity in the human brain. This research showed that the human brain retains the ability to generate new neurons throughout the lifetime (Eriksson, Perfilieva, Björk-Eriksson, Alborn, Nordborg, & Peterson, 1998). With neuroplasticity finally confirmed with the help of evidence from fMRI, the earlier work was given greater credence and paved the way for later research. It is now understood that the brain remains plastic and that we can work with this neuroplasticity (Harasym, 2008). It has also been shown that enriching environments result in improved brain function, making it reasonable to assume that functional recovery following TBI is possible.

Mechanisms of Neuroplasticity

Arden (2010) explains that the brain is constructed from millions of interconnected neurons that enable different tasks. One neuron is capable of connecting with as many as 10,000 other neurons, with new connections being formed as new tasks are learned. Connections are facilitated by neurotransmitters (brain chemicals) that carry messages across neurons at a junction known as the synapse. Stimulated neuronal pathways activate areas of the brain and create connections between multiple areas, increasing the overall capacity of the brain. The more often messages are carried across these pathways, the stronger the wiring becomes (Arden, 2010). Thus, the fundamental message of neuroplasticity is to activate the brain often (in the desired manner) to stimulate growth (Siegel, 2007). Conversely, if an area of the brain is not used the connections are likely to diminish over time.

Doidge (2010) described how neural pathways are built and how their function can be enhanced using the example of a tennis player. While any member of the general population can play tennis with varying degrees of competency, an elite tennis player develops extraordinary finesse and speed through hours of daily practice. Through repetition, the brain learns that this activity is important, and begins laying extra layers of myelin sheath (insulating material) on the neural pathways involved with performing the activity. The extra myelin transforms these nerve pathways into optimally conductive superhighways along which messages can move with greater frequency and speed. Interestingly, the speed with which these pathways are myelinated is increased when dopamine is released, which is more likely to occur in the presence of pleasure. Thus, brain development progresses well when the learning experience is pleasurable (Doidge, 2010). This capacity of the brain for continuous development means that healing and growth is something people can learn to harness. Not surprisingly, this message generated enormous hope and optimism among those with brain injury.

Neuroplasticity and Brain Injury

Neuroplasticity-based therapies offer promise for the treatment of the physical, cognitive, and psychosocial impacts of TBI from the time of injury and throughout recovery and rehabilitation. Research suggests that the brain may exhibit a heightened capacity for plasticity after injury, meaning structural and functional changes are more easily achieved than in the typical brain (Lillie & Mateer, 2011). However, plasticity is complex and is impacted by factors such as individual preexisting characteristics, time post injury, and the area injured (Raskin, 2011). Little is known about how these factors affect neuroplasticity, nor what interventions are most likely to be effective in promoting desired brain changes. Knowledge about the processes for best working with neuroplasticity for clinical applications is still in its infancy. Although some research has been conducted with those recovering from damage to the central nervous system, researchers are only just beginning to understand how to influence the mechanisms of neuroplasticity (DeFina et al., 2009; Young & Tolentino, 2011). DeFina et al. (2009) outlined a novel neuroplasticity-based treatment regime for TBI involving pharmaceutical and electromagnetic treatments tailored to individuals through the identification of specific neuromarkers. The aim of this treatment is to prevent the cascade of brain cell damage following brain injury, thus minimizing cell damage and enhancing cell repair. According to DeFina and colleagues, the new frontier of neuroplasticity will challenge our thinking about brain injury rehabilitation. The belief that recovery reaches a plateau at some point has been questioned, and there is now an incentive to explore interventions based on new understandings about neuroplasticity. Further, evidence suggests that clients can actively contribute to the ongoing design of the intervention based on their own experiences and observations, leading to the development of a self-managed repertoire of strategies, exercises and techniques. Collaboration between client and health professional at each new developmental stage has the potential to optimize benefits and minimize unintended outcomes.

As the potential for neuroplasticity to inform the rehabilitation and treatment of neurological disorders is now better understood, new techniques are being developed that can help to expedite recovery or maximize the surviving brain tissue (Young & Tolentino, 2011). The following sections outline the role of neuroplasticity in facilitating motor function, cognitive function, and mental health.

Harnessing Neuroplasticity to Improve Motor Function

Research on working with neuroplasticity has led to a range of innovative rehabilitation therapies that have relevance for people with TBI. For example a number of neuroplasticity-based rehabilitation approaches have been used to improve motor function following brain or spinal cord injury including constraint-induced movement therapy (CIMT), task-oriented physical therapy, and weight-supported treadmill training (Cramer et al., 2011). CIMT was pioneered by Edward Taub and colleagues at the University of Alabama to support people who have experienced stroke or traumatic brain injury in regaining the use of paralyzed limbs (see Taub & Wolf, 1997). CIMT is designed to enhance motor and functional recovery and involves restraining the functional limb throughout the day in order to re-train the affected limb (Young & Tolentino, 2011). Studies investigating the effect of CIMT on people following stroke demonstrated that the technique significantly improved motor function in the arm 3 to 9 months post stroke, compared to people who had not had the treatment (Sawaki et al., 2008; Wolf et al., 2006). In contrast with behavioral approaches, which use external aids to compensate for or substitute a lost function, these therapies aim to improve or restore the impaired function (Raskin, 2011). In relation to regaining lost function Raskin (2011) explains that plastic changes in the brain can involve either the healing of damaged areas, or another area taking on the task of the damaged part, and treatments must be designed with this distinction in mind. Restorative therapies are typically used in conjunction with other treatments including behavior-based therapies, and are often supported with meta-cognitive tools such as visualization.

Harnessing Neuroplasticity for Cognitive Rehabilitation

Cognitive therapies have been found to improve cognitive function for people with TBI, particularly in relation to activities concerned with attention, memory and executive function (Cicerone et al., 2005), which are typically challenging for people with TBI. Executive functioning has been defined as "the formation of intentions and programs, and the regulation and verification of activity" (Luria, 1973 cited in Hennessy, Geffen, Pauley, & Cutmore, 2003, p. 108). In relation to brain injury, cognitive rehabilitation can focus on either directly restoring lost connections, or on "reorganizing and re-distributing the cognitive workload" (Raskin, 2011, p. 110). Research using fMRI has provided visual evidence of brain plasticity in response to cognitive rehabilitation training for people with TBI (Kim et al., 2009; Laatsch et al., 2004). Results revealed a range of responses, reinforcing the notion that individualized programs are needed to optimize treatment effectiveness. A number of studies have looked at cognitive rehabilitation programs that were specifically designed to enhance neuroplasticity. One U.S. study investigated the efficacy of a novel neuroplasticity-based cognitive training program to improve memory in older adults (Smith et al., 2009). The experimental treatment involved a computerized neuroplasticity-based cognitive training program with exercises designed to enhance the accuracy and speed of auditory information processing. The exercises involved the acoustic organization of speech, and were based on the notion that improved sensory system function is related to improved cognitive function. The study found greater improvements in memory for the brain plasticity–based program than for the control group, who received a novelty and intensity-matched general stimulation program. Other studies have shown that neuroplasticity-based computerized cognitive rehabilitation training was effective in improving attention and memory functions (Lebowitz et al., 2009; Dams-O'Connor, Lebowitz, Cantor, & Spina, 2009).

Harnessing Neuroplasticity for Mental Health

Neuroplasticity also has relevance to the field of mental health, where early research suggests a relationship between brain plasticity and the ability to cope with stress and mental illness (Kays, Hurley, & Taber 2012). Neuroplasticity-based therapies are increasingly being used to treat a variety of mental health disorders such as depression, anxiety, phobias, post-traumatic stress disorder (PTSD) and obsessive compulsive disorder (OCD). One example of the therapeutic application of neuroplasticity for psychological disorders is the work of Schwartz and colleagues with recovery from OCD (Schwartz & Beyette, 1997; Schwartz & Begley; 2003). In the case of OCD, excessive thinking about a particular topic reinforces neural pathways in much the same way as the professional tennis player cultivated neural superhighways through repetitive physical actions. Research suggests that the greater the focus on a particular thought or behavior the more embedded it becomes in the neural network, increasing the likelihood of the thought or behavior being triggered (Schwartz & Begley, 2003). Ironically, therapies that focus on a specific problem could exacerbate that problem by strengthening the associated neural pathways.

Schwartz and colleagues investigated the brain mechanisms underlying OCD, and reasoned that a greater awareness in sufferers of these underlying mechanisms could increase their ability to control symptoms. Based on this premise, Schwartz designed a program of cognitive-behavioral therapy (CBT) using mindful attention. Through a process of *relabeling* and *reattributing* Schwartz guided people with OCD to view the condition as a brain glitch rather than an intrinsic element of self. Clients were shown their PET scans which demonstrated the neuroanatomical basis of the condition, and they were encouraged to observe their OCD with mindful awareness (i.e. experience their symptoms without judgment, and with the realization that symptoms were nothing more than a brain defect). This practice assisted people to relabel their obsession as a false signal. Schwartz further explained "through mindfulness, the patient distances himself (that is, his locus of conscious awareness) from his OCD (an intrusive experience entirely determined by material forces)" (Schwartz & Begley, 2003, p. 82). Clients directed their mental attention away from thoughts associated with OCD by *refocusing* on alternative, enjoyable behaviors, and were encouraged to *revalue* OCD by acknowledging that the obsession had no value and no intrinsic power. These active processes of *relabeling, reattributing, refocusing,* and *revaluing* changed the activation patterns of brain circuits, thereby directing neuroplasticity in desired directions and away from the obsessive behaviors. Based on the use it or lose it principle, Schwartz observed that the neural connections associated with the obsessive cycle began to diminish on PET scans and fMRI, but more importantly, new constructive pathways were being built, and the intensity of symptoms experienced by clients was reduced. Although the mechanisms underlying the relationship between neuroplasticity and mental health remain unclear, it seems multiple factors are involved, and further research is needed to inform treatments (Kays et al., 2012).

Using Mindfulness to Enhance Neuroplasticity

Schwartz's (Schwartz & Begley, 2003) work demonstrated the power of focused attention to alter brain circuits, habitual thoughts, and ultimately behavior, and is reflective of other mindfulness-based therapies. The practice of mindfulness has been described as a form of mental training that can induce neuroplasticity in positive directions (Davidson & Lutz, 2007). Mindfulness has been defined as "the awareness that emerges through paying attention on purpose, in the present moment, and non-judgmentally to the unfolding experience moment by moment" (Kabat-Zinn, 2003, p. 145). Although methods vary across programs, participants are typically guided to recognize their present physical and emotional experience, and to cultivate acceptance toward arising emotions or thoughts (Azulay, Mott, Cicerone, & Smart, 2012). The theory maintains that heightened awareness combined with acceptance leads to increased feelings of calm and well-being, and decreased feelings of anxiety and depression.

Mindfulness therapies are practices deriving from Buddhist meditation traditions, which have attracted increasing interest in recent years. Neuroimaging studies using electroencephalography (EEG) and fMRI have demonstrated neural changes in the brains of experienced meditators, revealing changes in brain structure in multiple brain regions compared to non-meditators (Lutz, Brefczynski-Lewis, Johnstone, & Davidson, 2008; Hölzel et al., 2008; Grant, Courtemanche, Duerden, Duncan, & Rainville, 2010). Similarly, studies of naïve meditators (i.e., those who had not practiced meditation before) taking part in eight-week mindfulness meditation courses have demonstrated changes in brain gray matter concentration (Hölzel et al., 2011) and in brain and immune function (Davidson et al., 2003). Results from another study showed that meditation was associated with increased activity in the left prefrontal cortex, an area of the brain associated with feelings of joy, happiness, and enthusiasm. Further, this area remained active after meditation had ceased, suggesting a long-term impact of meditation on brain functioning. At the same time, activity in the right prefrontal cortex, an area associated with feelings of depression and despair, became less active (Lutz, Brefczynski-Lewis, Johnstone, & Davidson, 2008).

Mindfulness-based interventions are increasingly being utilized in a range of clinical settings, and although methodological limitations have been noted, there is preliminary evidence attesting to the efficacy of such programs (Chiesa, Serretti, & Calati, 2011). For example mindfulness-based interventions have been shown to improve quality of life and well-being (Carmody & Baer, 2008), and to ameliorate symptoms associated with chronic pain (Grossman, Tiefenthaler-Gilmer, Raysz, & Kesper, 2007; Kabat-Zinn, Lipworth, & Burney, 1985), depression (Teasdale et al., 2000), anxiety (Evans et al., 2008), and stress associated with cancer (Speca, Carlson, Goodey, & Angen, 2000). The most widely used and researched programs in mainstream clinical and medical fields are mindfulness-based stress reduction (MBSR) (Kabat-Zinn, 1982, 1990) and mindfulness-based cognitive therapy (MBCT) (Teasdale et al., 2000; Segal, Williams, & Teasdale, 2002). MBSR was designed to assist the self-regulation of pain, and reduce stress for people with chronic pain or anxiety, while MBCT was originally used to prevent relapse of major depression. MBCT is based largely on the MBSR model, and incorporates cognitive therapy tools designed to facilitate detachment, or *decentering* from negative thoughts and emotions, thus "preventing the escalation of negative thoughts into ruminative patterns" (Baer, 2003, p. 127). Decentering or reperceiving describes the process of stepping back from the experience to shift cognitive sets to assume a more positive appraisal of the situation (Garland, Gaylord, & Park, 2008, p. 39). The same researchers suggest that decentering implicates second-order change in mental restructuring rather than first-order change where mental process rather than mental contents become the therapeutic focus.

Other models that reflect aspects of mindfulness training include acceptance and commitment therapy (ACT; Hayes, Strosahl, & Wilson, 2012), which teaches nonjudgmental acceptance; dialectical behaviour therapy (DBT; Linehan, 1993), which has been used to treat borderline personality disorder; and relapse prevention (RP; Marlatt & Gordon, 1985) a cognitive-behavioral intervention to prevent substance abuse relapse (Baer, 2003).

Mindfulness and Traumatic Brain Injury

Although evidence pointing to the efficacy of mindfulness-based interventions to treat a variety of conditions is increasing, only a few studies relate specifically to TBI. Results from non-TBI studies suggest that mindfulness interventions may help improve a range of symptoms typically associated with TBI including chronic pain, insomnia, affective disorders such as depression and anxiety, and cognitive impairments relating to attentional control, memory, and executive function (Azulay, Smart, Mott, & Cicerone, 2012; Bédard et al., 2012). Regions of the brain that have demonstrated morphological changes, suggesting improved function, after mindfulness training include the areas involved in learning and memory processes, perspective taking, emotional regulation, and self-referential processing (Hölzel et al., 2011). A meta-analysis of the effects of mindfulness-based therapy on anxiety and depression indicated that these therapies are promising for treating anxiety and mood problems in clinical populations (Hofmann, Sawyer, Witt, & Oh, 2010). Smaller effect sizes were found in another meta-analysis relating to the impact of mindfulness interventions on the mental health of people with a chronic illness (Bohlmeijer, Prenger, Taal, & Cuijpers, 2010). The authors of that study recommended the integration of mindfulness with cognitive behavioral therapies.

Despite the high incidence of depression and concomitant impaired concentration, mood swings, as well as reduced motivation experienced by people with TBI, these psychological and emotional problems often remain untreated (Bédard et al., 2012). As a response to this problem, Bédard and colleagues proposed a novel mindfulness-based intervention for people with TBI, which combined aspects of MBST, MBCT, breathing techniques, and yoga. Participants took part in an eight-week course that addressed topics including acceptance, present moment awareness, and awareness of thoughts and feelings. Results demonstrated that the intervention significantly reduced depression. The authors note the small scale of the study and lack of control group preclude the generalizability of the study, but results are promising, and suggest further larger scale trials are called for.

A systematic review of the impact of mindfulness training on cognitive abilities in healthy adults found that even brief mindfulness training improved sustained, selective, and executive attention, with long-term training resulting in further improvements, as well as indicating improvements in working memory (Chiesa et al., 2011). That mindfulness interventions have been shown to improve cognitive function and attention in healthy people does not necessarily mean that the same results will be reproduced for people with TBI. Indeed, mental and concentration activities have been associated with fatigue in people with TBI, suggesting mindfulness training may be difficult, or even detrimental for this population. Unrelated to injury severity, fatigue is a common long-term symptom of TBI and is associated with decreased neuronal efficiency, rather than a secondary symptom of pain, insomnia, or depression (Cantor et al., 2008). Interestingly, in one of the few studies of mindfulness and TBI, an investigation of the impact of a MBSR program on mental fatigue after stroke or TBI found significant improvements in fatigue on self-reports and neuropsychological tests (Johansson, Bjuhr, & Ronnback, 2012). The authors theorized that the intervention was helpful for people with TBI in that it promoted more efficient use of cognitive resources through stress reduction strategies, which in turn reduced mental fatigue. Over the course of the program participants became less tired during sessions, and the inclusion of a physical component in the form of yoga helped facilitate focused attention.

Property oᵢ
Baker College
of Allen Park

Azulay and colleagues (2012) reasoned, "given that attention is one set of cognitive functions shown to be amenable to cognitive rehabilitation, one might then extrapolate that mindfulness training could impact attention in individuals for whom this ability is impaired" (p. 2). Following from this, a pilot study was carried out to examine the effect of a ten-week MBSR program on the chronic symptoms associated with mild TBI including cognitive symptoms such as reduced attention, mental control, and executive dysfunction; physical symptoms, such as headache, sensory changes, and cognitive/physical fatigue; psychiatric sequelae, including depression, anxiety, and post traumatic stress disorder (PTST); and emotional dysregulation. Results indicated improvements in quality of life measures, perceived self-efficacy, and the central executive aspects of working memory and attention. As a result of mindfulness training, participants' ability to monitor and manage stress improved, and perhaps more importantly, participants gained the sense that they were in control and able to manage their own symptoms (Azulay et al., 2012). It should be noted that mindfulness programs can be modified for people with TBI to take account of cognitive impairments. Techniques such as shortened sessions, the use of memory aids, and repetition, and frequent reviews can all assist people with TBI to undertake mindfulness training (Bédard et al., 2012). Unlike traditional rehabilitation programs that emphasize improvement or behavior change, mindfulness practice emphasizes an absence of striving or force, which may be particularly helpful for people with TBI.

A Novel Therapy Using Biofeedback to Support Mindfulness and Promote Neuroplasticity

A neuro-rehabilitation technique that can help people intentionally direct neuroplasticity toward desirable outcomes, and can be used to support mindfulness training, is biofeedback. Biofeedback is a therapeutic process used to improve mental health and well-being, involving the real-time feedback of physiological information to clients. Measurements such as heart rate, muscle tension, and temperature are "fed back" to people, allowing them to monitor and self-regulate these physiological factors. The presentation of this information makes tangible the reciprocal relationship between cognitive and physiological processes, and allows people "to be actively involved in the control of their own physiological and emotional processes" (Myers and Young, 2012). The inclusion of biofeedback in mindfulness practice assists people to maintain focus and present moment awareness, and could be a helpful adjunct to mindfulness training for people with TBI.

Biofeedback is a well-established treatment with demonstrated efficacy for reducing symptoms in a range of disorders including autism spectrum disorder (Coben, Linden, & Myers, 2010; Naser et al., 2012), posttraumatic stress disorder (PTSD; Sherlin, Arns, Lubar, & Sokhadze,

2010), drug addiction (Sokhadze, Stewart, & Hollifield, 2007), attention-deficit/hyperactivity disorder (ADHD; Arns, deRidder, Stehrl, Breteler, & Cohen, 2009), and anxiety and depression (Myers & Young, 2012). Research has shown that neurofeedback (a form of biofeedback) is particularly effective for treating inattention and impulsivity in people with ADHD (Arns et al., 2009). However, its use as a treatment intervention in facilitating self-awareness following brain injury is limited. One study (Ackerman, 2004) has explored the potential of biofeedback in clients with both TBI and PTSD. Although based on single case study data, results of this work provide evidence of increased self-control of blood pressure, decreased frequency of negative thoughts, moderated depressed feelings, elimination of headaches and nightmares and decreased panic (Ackerman, 2004).

The following section describes a novel dual neurorehabilitation intervention treatment program based on mindfulness and biofeedback currently being used at the York Mind-Body Health Centre, UK, which could have fruitful application to TBI rehabilitation. The center is a newly developed psychological treatment service located at York University. The program involves mindfulness training using a neurophysiological intervention (neurofeedback) in combination with a behavioral intervention of cognitive awareness training (acceptance and commitment therapy [ACT]), as a way of managing recognized psychological disorders such as panic attacks, anxiety, and phobias, and for managing chronic pain. Although not specifically oriented to traumatic brain injury clients, the combined therapeutic approach represents an innovative way to approach brain injury rehabilitation, particularly in relation to hard to manage awareness deficits and difficult to engage clients. Each intervention is the subject of advanced practice in its own right, however, the benefits of employing a combined therapeutic approach in brain injury using ACT has been previously confirmed (see Kangas & McDonald, 2011).

The combined approach offered by the York service suggests that in neuro-feedback physiological parameters that correlate with subjective experience are measured. This information is fed back in real time, typically via computer monitoring. The instant client feedback creates an opportunity for enhanced awareness of the interrelationships between people's thoughts, emotions, and physiology, and the power of one's intention to accept and influence these factors. Based on this awareness people can learn to influence their physiological state in a direction more favorable to positive mental states (Blackett, 2011, personal communication). The most expedient and useful biofeedback parameters are those that are easy to measure, have a clearly recognizable relationship to subjective experience, and are relatively easy to control, including parameters such as electromyography (EMG) as an indicator of muscle tension; heart rate coherence (HRC) as an indicator of synchronization between breathing and heart rate; and infrared (IR) temperature as an indicator of brain metabolic activity. Some key mechanisms of change of biofeedback and cognitive acceptance are outlined below:

* Biofeedback gives clients direct insight into the mind–body connection, and especially that their thoughts give rise to bodily responses, both pleasant and unpleasant.
* Biofeedback helps clients master the art of cognitive decentering. They learn to embody the process as a reduction of muscle tension — literally letting go.
* Biofeedback helps clients master the art of acceptance. It demonstrates the reality of being in the present and how inner resistance and struggle can serve to amplify problems.
* Biofeedback can assist clients' motivation to maintain a regular mindfulness meditation practice simply by making it easier and more engaging.
* Biofeedback can support the development of "emotional intelligence" — how emotions are mind–body phenomena that can be monitored and managed.

Conclusion

Current understandings suggest that interventions aiming to harness neuroplasticity for recovery after TBI need to be intense, frequent, and include a variety of cognitive and physical therapies (Kolb et al., 2011). However, a greater understanding of the complexities of neuroplasticity is needed before optimal treatments can be identified. Cramer et al. (2011) notes possible directions for future research including individualized treatments based on client measurements such as functional status and residual brain circuits, the examination of therapies in combination, and a greater understanding of treatment mechanisms at every level. Once these mechanisms of neuroplasticity become clear, sophisticated intervention techniques are likely to emerge, experimental techniques are likely to become more widely available and strategies drawing on neuroplasticity will likely become embedded into the rehabilitation process. Research on the application of techniques to work with neuroplasticity, specifically to repair functions affected by brain injury, is in its early stages. However, there are many things people with TBI can begin to do to enhance their well-being, and minimize the risk of depression. Mindfulness and biofeedback could offer some people with TBI useful tools to capitalize on neuroplasticity.

References

Ackerman, R. J. (2004). Applied psychophysiology, clinical biofeedback, and rehabilitation neuropsychology: a case study — mild traumatic brain injury and post-traumatic stress disorder. *Physical Medicine and Rehabilitation Clinics of North America, 15*(4), 919–931.

Arden, J. B. (2010). *Rewire your brain: Think your way to a better life*. New Jersey: John Wiley.

Arns, M., de Ridder, S., Strehl, U., Breteler, M., & Coenen, A. (2009). Efficacy of neurofeedback treatment in ADHD: the effects on inattention, impulsivity and hyperactivity: a meta-analysis. *Clinical EEG and Neuroscience: Official Journal of the EEG and Clinical Neuroscience Society (ENCS), 40*(3), 180.

Arrowsmith-Young, B. (2012). *The woman who changed her brain: and other inspiring stores of pioneering brain transformation*. New York: Free Press.

Azulay, J., Smart, C. M., Mott, T., & Cicerone, K. D. (2012). A pilot study examining the effect of mindfulness-based stress reduction on symptoms of chronic mild traumatic brain injury/postconcussive syndrome. *Journal of Head Trauma Rehabilitation*, 1–9.

Baer, R. A. (2003). Mindfulness training as a clinical intervention: a conceptual and empirical review. *Clinical Psychology: Science and Practice, 10*(2), 125–143.

Bédard, M., Felteau, M., Marshall, S., Dubois, S., Gibbons, C., Klein, R., & Weaver, B. (2012). Mindfulness-based cognitive therapy: benefits in reducing depression following a traumatic brain injury. *Advances in Mind–Body Medicine, 26*(1), 14.

Bohlmeijer, E., Prenger, R., Taal, E., & Cuijpers, P. (2010). The effects of mindfulness-based stress reduction therapy on mental health of adults with a chronic medical disease: a meta-analysis. *Journal of Psychosomatic Research, 68*(6), 539–544.

Cantor, J. B., Ashman, T., Gordon, W., Ginsberg, A., Engmann, C., Egan, M., & Flanagan, S. (2008). Fatigue after traumatic brain injury and its impact on participation and quality of life. *The Journal of Head Trauma Rehabilitation, 23*(1), 41–51.

Carmody, J., & Baer, R. A. (2008). Relationships between mindfulness practice and levels of mindfulness, medical and psychological symptoms and well-being in a mindfulness-based stress reduction program. *Journal of Behavioral Medicine, 31*(1), 23–33.

Chiesa, A., Serretti, A., & Calati, R. (2011). Does mindfulness training improve cognitive abilities? A systematic review of neuropsychological findings. *Clinical Psychology Review, 31*(3), 449–464.

Cicerone, K. D., Dahlberg, C., Malec, J. F., Langenbahn, D. M., Felicetti, T., Kneipp, S., & Catanese, J. (2005). Evidence-based cognitive rehabilitation: Updated review of the literature from 1998 through 2002. *Archives of Physical Medicine and Rehabilitation, 86*(8), 1681–1692.

Coben, R., Linden, M., & Myers, T. E. (2010). Neurofeedback for autistic spectrum disorder: a review of the literature. *Applied Psychophysiology and Biofeedback, 35*(1), 83–105.

Cramer, S. C., Sur, M., Dobkin, B. H., O'Brien, C., Sanger, T. D., Trojanowski, J. Q., & Vinogradov, S. (2011). Harnessing neuroplasticity for clinical applications. *Brain: a Journal of Neurology, 134*(Pt 6), 1591–1609.

Dams-O'Connor, K., Lebowitz, M., Cantor, J., & Spina, L. (2009). *Feasibility of a computerized cognitive skill-building program in an inpatient TBI rehabilitation setting*. Poster presented at the American Congress of Rehabilitation Medicine, Denver, CO.

Davidson, R. J., Kabat-Zinn, J., Schumacher, J., Rosenkranz, M., Muller, D., Santorelli, S. F., & Sheridan, J. F. (2003). Alterations in brain and immune function produced by mindfulness meditation. *Psychosomatic Medicine, 65*(4), 564–570.

Davidson, R. J., & Lutz, A. (2007). Buddha's brain: Neuroplasticity and meditation. *IEEE Signal Processing Magazine, 25*(1), 176–174.

DeFina, P. Fellus, J. ZemyanPolito, M. Thompson, J.W.G. Scolaro Moser, R. De-Luca, J. (2009): The new neuroscience frontier: Promoting neuroplasticity and brain repair in traumatic brain injury, *The Clinical Neuropsychologist, 23*(8), 1391–1399.

Doidge, N. (2010). *The brain that changes itself: Stories of personal triumph from the frontiers of brain science.* Melbourne: Scribe Publications.

Eriksson, P. S., Perfilieva, E., Björk-Eriksson, T., Alborn, A. M., Nordborg, C., & Peterson, D. A. (1998). Neurogenesis in the adult human hippocampus. *Nature Medicine, 4*(11), 1313–1317.

Evans, S., Ferrando, S., Findler, M., Stowell, C., Smart, C., & Haglin, D. (2008) Mindfulness-based cognitive therapy for generalized anxiety disorder. *Journal of Anxiety Disorders, 22,* 716–721.

Garland, E., Gaylord, S., & Park, J. (2009). The role of mindfulness in positive re-appraisal. *Explore: The Journal of Science and Healing, 5*(1), 37–44.

Grant, J. A., Courtemanche, J., Duerden, E. G., Duncan, G. H., & Rainville, P. (2010). Cortical thickness and pain sensitivity in zen meditators. *Emotion, 10*(1), 43–53.

Grossman, P., Tiefenthaler-Gilmer, U., Raysz, A., & Kesper, U. (2007). Mindfulness training as an intervention for fibromyalgia: Evidence of postintervention and 3-year follow-up benefits in well-being. *Psychotherapy and psychosomatics, 76*(4), 226–233.

Harasym, P. H. (2008). Neuroplasticity and critical thinking. *The Kaohsiung Journal of Medical Sciences, 24*(7), 339–340.

Hayes, S. C., Strosahl, K., & Wilson, K. G. (2012). *Acceptance and commitment therapy: the process and practice of mindful change.* New York: Guilford Press.

Hebb, D. O. (1949). *The organization of behavior: a neuropsychological theory.* New York: Wiley.

Hennessy, M. J., Geffen, G., Pauley, G., & Cutmore, T. (2003) The assessment of executive functioning following mild traumatic brain injury. *Brain Impairment, 4*(2), 106–121.

Hofmann, S. G., Sawyer, A. T., Witt, A. A., & Oh, D. (2010). The effect of mindfulness-based therapy on anxiety and depression: a meta-analytic review. *Journal of Consulting Clinical Psychology, 78*(2), 169–183.

Hölzel, B. K., Carmody, J., Vangel, M., Congleton, C., Yerramsetti, S. M., Gard, T., & Lazar, S. W. (2011). Mindfulness practice leads to increases in regional brain gray matter density. *Psychiatry Research, 191*(1), 36–43.

Hölzel, B. K., Ott, U., Gard, T., Hempel, H., Weygandt, M., Morgen, K., & Vaitl, D. (2008). Investigation of mindfulness meditation practitioners with voxel-based morphometry. *Social Cognitive and Affective Neuroscience, 3*(1), 55–61.

Johansson, B., Bjuhr, H., & Ronnback, L. (2012). Mindfulness-based stress reduction (MBSR)—a promising treatment for long-term mental fatigue after traumatic brain injury or stroke. *Brain Injury, 26*(4), 1–8.

Kabat-Zinn, J. (1982). An outpatient program in behavioral medicine for chronic pain patients based on the practice of mindfulness meditation: Theoretical considerations and preliminary results. *General Hospital Psychiatry, 4,* 33–47.

Kabat-Zinn, J. (1990). *Full catastrophe living: using the wisdom of your body and mind to face stress, pain and illness.* New York: Delacorte.

Kabat-Zinn, J. (2003). Mindfulness-based interventions in context: past, present, and future. *Clinical Psychology: Science and Practice, 10*(2), 144–156.

Kabat-Zinn, J., Lipworth, L., & Burney, R. (1985). The clinical use of mindfulness meditation for the self-regulation of chronic pain. *Journal of Behavioral Medicine, 8,* 163–190.

Kangas, M., & McDonald, S. (2011). Is it time to act? The potential of acceptance and commitment therapy for psychological problems following acquired brain injury. *Neuropsychological Rehabilitation: An International Journal, 21*(2), 250–276.

Kays, J. L., Hurley, R. A., & Taber, K. H. (2012). The dynamic brain: neuroplasticity and mental health. *Journal of Neuropsychiatry and Clinical Neurosciences, 24*(2), 118–124.

Kim, Y.-H., Yoo, W.-K., Ko, M.-H., Park, C.-h., Kim, S. T., & Na, D. L. (2009). Plasticity of the attentional network after brain injury and cognitive rehabilitation. *Neurorehabilitation and Neural Repair, 23*(5), 468–477.

Kolb, B., Muhammad, A., & Gibb, R. (2011). Searching for factors underlying cerebral plasticity in the normal and injured brain. *Journal of Communication Disorders, 44*(5), 503–514.

Laatsch, L. K., Thulborn, K. R., Krisky, C. M., Shobat, D. M., & Sweeney, J. A. (2004). Investigating the neurobiological basis of cognitive rehabilitation therapy with fMRI. *Brain Injury, 18*(10), 957–974.

Lebowitz, M., Cantor, J., Dams-O'Connor, K., Ashman, T., Tsaousides, T., Gordon, W., et al. (2009). *Examining the usability of a computerized cognitive training program in people with traumatic brain injury (TBI): A pilot study.* Poster presented at the American Congress of Rehabilitation Medicine, Denver, CO.

Lillie, R. A., & Mateer, C. A. Neuroplasticity and the treatment of executive deficits: Conceptual considerations. In Raskin S. A. (Ed). *Neuroplasticity and rehabilitation,* (pp. 257–284). New York: Guilford Press.

Linehan, M. M. (1993). Dialectical behavior therapy for treatment of borderline personality disorder: implications for the treatment of substance abuse. *NIDA Research Monograph, 137,* 201.

Lutz, A., Brefczynski-Lewis, J., Johnstone, T., & Davidson, R. J. (2008) Regulation of the neural circuitry of emotion by compassion meditation: effects of meditative expertise. *PLoS One 3*(3), e1897.

Marlatt, G.A., & Gordon, J.R., eds. (1985). *Relapse prevention: Maintenance strategies in the treatment of addictive behaviors.* New York: Guilford Press.

Myers, J. E., & Young, J. S. (2012). Brain wave biofeedback: Benefits of integrating neurofeedback in counseling. *Journal of Counseling and Development, 90*(1), 20.

Naser, M., Thomas, M., Richard, B., Christine, K., Lutz, W., Michael, R., et al. (2012). Combining biofeedback and narrative exposure therapy for persistent pain and PTSD in refugees: a pilot study. *European Journal of Psychotraumatology, 3,* 1–6.

Raskin, S. A. (2011). *Neuroplasticity and rehabilitation.* New York: Guilford Press.

Sawaki, L., Butler, A. J., Leng, X., Wassenaar, P. A., Mohammad, Y. M., Blanton, S., & Wittenberg, G. F. (2008). Constraint-induced movement therapy results in increased motor map area in subjects 3 to 9 months after stroke. *Neurorehabilitation and Neural Repair, 22*(5), 505–513.

Schwartz, J. M., & Begley, S. (2003) *The mind and the brain: Neuroplasticity and the power of mental force.* New York: Harper Perennial.

Schwartz, J. M., & Beyette, B. (1997) *Free yourself from obsessive-compulsive behavior: A four-step self-treatment method to change your brain chemistry.* New York: Regan Books.

Segal, Z. V., Williams, J. M. G., & Teasdale, J. D. (2002). *Mindfulness-based cognitive therapy for depression: A new approach to preventing relapse.* New York: Guilford Press.

Sherlin, L., Arns, M., Lubar, J., & Sokhadze, E. (2010). A position paper on neurofeedback for the treatment of ADHD. *Journal of Neurotherapy, 14*(2), 66–78.

Siegel, D. J. (2007) The mindful brain: Reflection and attunement in the cultivation of well-being New York, London: W. W. Norton.

Smith, G. E., Housen, P., Yaffe, K., Ruff, R., Kennison, R. F., Mahncke, H. W., & Zelinski, E. M. (2009). A cognitive training program based on principles of brain plasticity: Results from the Improvement in Memory with Plasticity-based Adaptive Cognitive Training (IMPACT) study. *Journal of the American Geriatrics Society, 57*(4), 594–603.

Sokhadze, T., Stewart, C., & Hollifield, M. (2007). Integrating cognitive neuroscience research and cognitive behavioral treatment with neurofeedback therapy in drug addiction comorbid with posttraumatic stress disorder: a conceptual review. *Journal of Neurotherapy, 11*(2), 13–44.

Speca, M., Carlson, L. E., Goodey, E., & Angen, M. (2000). A randomized, wait-list controlled clinical trial: the effect of a mindfulness meditation-based stress reduction program on mood and symptoms of stress in cancer outpatients. *Psychosomatic Medicine, 62*(5), 613.

Taub, E., & Wolf, S.L. (1997). Constraint-induced (CI) movement techniques to facilitate upper extremity use in stroke patients. *Topics in Stroke Rehabilitation,* 3, 38–61.

Teasdale, J. D., Segal, Z. V., Williams, J. M. G., Ridgeway, V. A., Soulsby, J. M., & Lau, M. A. (2000). Prevention of relapse/recurrence in major depression by mindfulness-based cognitive therapy. *Journal of Consulting and Clinical Psychology, 68*(4), 615–623.

Wolf, S. L., Winstein, C. J., Miller, J. P., Taub, E., Uswatte, G., Morris, D., & EXCITE Investigators. (2006). Effect of constraint-induced movement therapy on upper extremity function 3 to 9 months after stroke: the EXCITE randomized clinical trial. *JAMA, 296*(17), 2095–2104.

Young, J. A., & Tolentino, M. (2011). Neuroplasticity and its applications for rehabilitation. *American Journal of Therapeutics, 18*(1), 70–80.

CHAPTER 3

The Subtlety of Brain Injury: Surviving and Thriving through Playfulness

Susan Wenberg

My friend Bill truthfully states that he is an excellent computer programmer. He reminds me that his superior performance is not because he is brilliant—he is—but so are all his coworkers. Bill excels at his work because he is also an excellent typist. He tells me he can type as fast as he thinks. The ability to type rapidly, combined with brilliance and training, yield an excellent computer programmer.

I found Bill's story touching because I am a poor typist. I realize I am intelligent and could be trained as a computer programmer, but I cannot even imagine typing quickly. Difficulty with typing, writing, running, and a host of motor-skill activities has been my legacy since I sustained a head injury 30 years ago. I am one of many who have experienced the subtle but profound changes that follow a head injury. Since my injury I have completed a doctorate of chiropractic degree as well as a master's degree, successfully run a business, treated thousands of patients, and published journal articles. My injury has not prevented me from accomplishing these tasks, but it has adversely impacted my life, altered my career, and made simple daily activities difficult—difficult enough that I have spent a substantial amount of my time and energy embracing rehabilitative efforts.

In this chapter I share some personal and clinical experiences that demonstrate the subtle expressions of brain injury, and a few thoughts about remediation. These subtle consequences of head injury may remain unrecognized and untreated because the clinical focus is on the more serious components. When there is no serious component, the subtle component of head injury may not even be recognized.

I prefer the term "subtle" rather than "mild" as the impact is far from mild. Changes in perception, organization, energy, and personality may be described as subtle, but they play havoc with an individual's life, particularly if the signs are misinterpreted or not identified. Our ability to organize ourselves in our environment, and rely on our perceptions and energy levels, influence how we interact with family members, coworkers, and the world around us.

Our personal character traits—those traits that distinguish us from colleagues and friends, those that prompted our spouse to marry us rather than someone else—are more changeable than we like to imagine. We tend to think of our personality as permanent, yet when we see loved ones with dementia or progressive neurological loss, we see their personalities altered over time. A brain injury can alter a personality in a moment. Subtle changes in personality and executive function might always be noticed by coworkers, friends, and family, and sometimes by the injured individual. Often, however, the changes are not attributed to neurological insult, nor are they addressed clinically. There are multiple reasons for the misinterpretation of these subtle changes. None of us truly know how others perceive the world therefore we are not well positioned to know if that perception has changed. Perception is subconscious, so unless someone we know is suddenly walking into walls, or no longer recognizes us, we and they may not be aware of their subtle perceptual changes.

All of us experience fluctuations in our energy level and ability to organize. We attribute those fluctuations to stress, poor sleep, or some other temporal factor. It would be human nature to attribute such losses to factors with which we are already familiar rather than to a brain injury. Brain injuries manifest differently in different people because individuals are unique and because there are countless variations of brain injury. There are fewer measurable clinical guideposts for subtle perceptual and behavioral changes in comparison to, say, paralysis or sensory loss. There is no universal paradigm for understanding these subtle changes. In brain injury, there is a tendency to explain and justify what we see using well-used paradigms, attributing changes to stress, medication, inherent poor coordination, or a bad day, rather than something organic and much more complex such as TBI, thus missing opportunities for appropriate remediation. The subtle nature of TBI also means that we may have lost skills and abilities we didn't even know we had. For example, I drove across the United States many times in the five years following my head injury—always safely. I positioned myself behind a commercial cargo truck, and followed that truck for hours, keeping a safe distance and changing lanes whenever the truck driver did. I considered it a brilliant strategy because truck drivers in the United States are generally safe and well-informed.

It seemed to me that following a truck driver lowered my risk of getting a speeding ticket. However, there was another reason I linked my behavior with a truck driver's behavior, one that took me a dozen years to fully comprehend: I simply could not maintain a consistent speed without the guidance of the truck in front.

Years later I grasped the concept that intrinsic rhythm was an ability that can be lost after brain injury. I had joined a swim team, where my left-sided weakness haunted me at every workout, as it does to this day. I failed to realize that I could not maintain a steady pace in the pool, nor could I sense my gradual changes in speed. I had success with drum lessons as an adolescent and had assumed I was expressing a sense of rhythm that was inherent to human nature. Therefore, I considered the later fluctuations in my ability to maintain swimming and driving speeds as anomalies. Since I could not even perceive gradual changes in acceleration or deceleration, the changes in my ability did not seem real to me. It did not match my physical experience, driving history, or perception of myself, built in the years before my injury. My inability to hold pace had not been evident during years of postinjury urban driving where frequent stops and changes in speed are the norm. I attributed my erratic swimming speed to my physical weakness, starting at an inappropriate pace or simply daydreaming while swimming. I was missing the one critical piece that would have allowed me to identify my loss: a paradigm in which rhythm is linked to neurological function that could be lost or altered. I had always known that some kids had a better sense of rhythm than I, and some kids had no sense of rhythm. I knew my sense was adequate for my needs and I never thought about it again. I had no idea my sense of rhythm could change, even when it did.

It was through a course in neurological rehabilitation where I identified my loss of rhythm and then sought remediation. Now, years later, I drive hundreds of miles each month, at a consistent speed and without relying on a truck driver. I swim at a consistent pace, if I am prudent enough to pick a pace that matches my energy level. However, neurological recovery is not linear in its expression or in its persistence. When I have overstressed my neurological system, fatigue sets in and rhythm eludes me. When that happens I slip behind a truck driver, or another swimmer in my lane, reverting to my old strategies.

This example from my life illustrates why individuals with brain injuries are often hypervigilant; they cannot rely on their subconscious self to guide actions such as turning off the burner on the stove after cooking, taking everything they need when leaving for work, getting to the airport on time for a flight, or stopping at a stop light. When reaching for a glass of water perhaps they cannot safely predict that they will grasp the glass without knocking it over.

One of my patients succinctly described his personal experience with a subtle brain injury: "The things about myself I like the most I cannot even find, and the things I have always hated about myself are with me all the time." Another patient described a trip to the grocery store. He purchased everything he intended, but upon returning home placed the perishables in the laundry hamper rather than the refrigerator. It was several days before he noticed the mistake. Yet another patient described how she would get lost when driving between work and home, although she had traversed that route hundreds of times. Once she realized where she was, she had to determine what her intentions had been; was she driving to work? going home from work? or going to the grocery store? One patient called me to see if she was scheduled for an appointment in my office that day. When I replied in the affirmative, she asked if she had already been to it or was it still pending. It is not surprising that these "software glitches" affect our ability to navigate our world and manage our relationships. It is unsettling for all involved.

Brain injuries are like tornadoes; they arrive with very little warning, and destroy portions of the landscape while inexplicably leaving other portions untouched. No tornado is exactly like another, nor does a tornado destroy identical functions in different cities.

I find it interesting that I can still draw complex metabolic pathways from memory, effectively debate both sides of a complicated argument, make complex medical decisions, design databases and three dimensional structures, and yet have trouble dancing a waltz or accurately dialing a phone number. I can conceptualize what my legs, arms, and eyes should do, but I can't always get my body to cooperate. My poor coordination expresses itself in simple acts, such as typing, running, and reading. It took me years to embrace my physical endeavors from the perspective of neurological function rather than physical exercise. Now I exercise with a primary goal of neurological enhancement, and a secondary goal of physical fitness.

I am grateful that my intellectual ability was not impacted by my injury, because my sense of identity is strongly linked to my intellectual self. However, my capacity to express that intellect in the community was impaired. Speaking and writing have been burdensome following my injury. Five years following my injury, I finished my graduate level written exams long before I had completed everything I wanted to say; I stopped when I could no longer write. I made the mistake of sharing this observation with my colleagues. Without the paradigm for understanding my action, they interpreted it as disrespectful and foolish. Their understanding was incorrect, but I could not offer a better one.

Denial after Brain Injury

I am often amused by the statements of middle-aged patients who come into my office with pain syndromes that are clearly related to their age and poor physical condition. They ask me, "How could this happen to me? I am a great athlete. I was a star baseball player in high school."

I ask myself, "don't they realize that was 30 years ago when they weighed 80 pounds less? Don't they see their current self when they look in the mirror?"

I am less amused when I am confronted by similar misperceptions in my own body. I much prefer the image of myself when I was 22: when I had a normal and symmetrical level of coordination and strength; when my left side worked as well as my right; when I could stand or read for long periods of time without fatigue. I have come to realize that it is human nature to identify with our preferred self—the self who performed well and who never imagined that the ability to perform was transient. Losing function as one gets older, or for any other reason, is threatening. Denial is a natural response.

Denial on the part of the patient or the family is generally considered to be detrimental. However, I have seen that denial serves a protective role when the impact of the brain injury is just too much for the patient or family to embrace. Paradoxically, subtle symptoms can be more disruptive to one's sense of self than overt symptoms. Individuals with these so-called minor losses may be more disturbed by their losses than individuals with severe loss. It seems far more difficult to accept subtle change in ourselves and the people we love. I have learned that a little misperception can be good for our soul. It gives us the spirit to keep going, and to confront tasks that might seem overwhelming if we were more realistic.

Playfulness

In the small liberal arts college where I earned my undergraduate education, it was customary for the students in the women's dormitory to host a "Screw Your Roommate" dance, where each woman was in charge of finding a date for their roommate. Not all roommates were the best of friends, so it is understandable that the days leading up to the dance were fraught with trepidation and sometimes sabotage. Anxiety was the norm, but there was one component of this event that was anxiety free: asking a gorgeous guy for a date. There was no risk to the asker's personal identity, as the woman was not asking for a date for herself but for her roommate. Securing a date was like a game; failure or success, they both felt safe. Contrast this with seriously asking someone for a date when rejection would seem like a personal failure, or a threat to one's sense of self. By designing a situation (albeit, in this case unconventional to say the least) where asking for a date was safe, the action moves from one of threat to one of playful enthusiasm.

At a broader level there is richness in embracing any venture, including dating or neurological rehabilitation, as though it were a game. Business coaches encourage the work as play model, and educators use games to teach students skills and comprehension. In a similar manner, play is an ideal context for our rehabilitation efforts. Play is an ideal medium for developing a helpful emotional tone. Play encourages us to push beyond our emotional and physical boundaries—safely.

> Confronting one's neurological losses is not fun whereas play is fun.
> Work is drudgery, but play is entertaining.
> Losing at life is devastating, but losing at play is something we have all experienced and survived.

I often apply the concept of play in my clinical practice, and in my life—including the subset of my life that is an ongoing rehabilitation journey. For instance, my loss of coordination is reflected in my speech, or perhaps I should say, used to be reflected in my speech. I have often embraced formal rehabilitation protocols, but it does get tiring. I wanted neurological improvement, but I wanted a break from working on my head injury. I considered speech therapy, but felt burdened by the therapy concept. What to do? In a moment of creativity, I opted for private singing lessons. I had learned that I was tone deaf in first grade. I also knew that one makes one's greatest gains when addressing one's weakest areas. Singing lessons seemed like the perfect fit. Being exposed as tone deaf was not threatening to me because the ability to carry a tune was not part of my 22-year-old, preinjury identity. I met with my voice instructor once a week, never practicing between sessions; I could not tell whether I was singing in tune, so what was the point of practicing without her feedback?

Neurological progress is not linear. While driving down the road one day after almost a year of lessons I spontaneously sang one of my favorite Taize chants. I knew intrinsically that I had started on the correct note and had been reasonably accurate during the rest of the chant. No one was more surprised than me, except perhaps my instructor. Voice lessons taught me many things, for example tone deafness is a myth. Also, Arias can be much more difficult than they seem!

More importantly, I learned to shape my mouth and tongue in ways I never knew existed, and to produce sounds I could never imagine producing. It was hard work because I could not conceptualize what was required to create a specific sound or hit a certain note. At the same time it was fun precisely because it was experiential rather than conceptual, and because I didn't particularly care about success. I didn't really want to be able sing; but now I can. More importantly, my speech is clearer, I no longer gag when drinking or eating, and I notice spillover improvement in swimming and bicycling. I also have a greater appreciation for music and musicians. For the first time, I find myself intrigued by opera.

In a similar manner, I struggled for years to improve my lack of organizational or efficiency skills e—both those inherent to my nature and those unique to my head injury. Efficiency (or organization) had eluded me, and I knew it. An astute business coach helped me identify something else that had eluded me; coziness. She wisely encouraged me to direct my attention toward the experience of coziness rather than efficiency. I had enjoyed many pleasurable experiences over the prior 25 years, but they were intellectual observations of pleasure. I could not quite feel them physically. I could not savor them. I had lost my sense of coziness, but was unable to define its absence. Physical discomfort, but more than that—a sense of disconnect—factored into my loss, the disconnect between my preinjury and postinjury life, the disconnect between my perception of my body and the way it actually moved, the disconnect between different parts of myself—a disconnect that was not there before.

I simply could not feel physically comfortable. I was tired yet unsettled; sleepy yet vigilant. My cat is incredibly vigilant, yet she relaxes better than anyone I know. I was missing the relaxing part. I would sleep for 15 hours yet awaken unrefreshed. I didn't know how to do, feel, or move comfortably. I was missing the comfortable feeling of coziness. Over the years I have regained a feeling of coziness. Sometimes I experience just a shadow of it. On a good day, I am in the same league as my cat.

Three Concepts in Neurological Rehabilitation

Now, after 20 years of experience as a practitioner, I serve my patients more effectively than I did as a new physician. I simply know more: intellectually, perceptually, and experientially. Based on that knowledge, I can share three concepts that embody my perceptual and experiential understanding of rehabilitation following brain injury.

The Metabolic Threshold

The goal of rehabilitation is to craft a brain that is efficient and flexible as well as strong. Neurological fatigue is not like nudging the boundaries of physical exertion—overdoing it has adverse consequences. It is best to use caution when nearing the level of neurological fatigue. For instance, the one-hour sessions supported by clinics and hospitals may be far more than a patient can neurologically endure at one time.

There is a term black hole day in the brain injury community: a day when all one's efforts produce no results—when coordination, energy, and organized thought take a holiday. It is similar to the experience of trying to drive a car when there is no gas in the tank: everything looks like it should work but it doesn't work at all. Athletes call it "hitting the wall." Chiropractic neurologists call it "exceeding the metabolic threshold." It happens when the individual's neurological system runs out of gas. The individual is no longer able to perform. In vulnerable individuals, exceeding the metabolic threshold can trigger a seizure or migraine. Unfortunately, it does not take a marathon athletic event to exceed the metabolic threshold of a compromised individual. The noisy or visually stimulating environment of a restaurant, store, or workplace might be enough to overload the system.

The key to rehabilitation is knowing how much and what type of stimulus to apply, while honoring the need for down time. Rest, sleep, and quiet time are necessary to integrate the stimulus provided by therapy. Once formal rehabilitation has come to an end, it is up to the injured individual and family to keep stimulus at an appropriate level and to respect down time.

Relaxation

There is a concept in neurology that a relaxed body is a reflection of an intact and well-functioning brain. For those of us raised with a puritan work ethic, this concept may seem counterintuitive or downright immoral. For those of us who find it difficult to relax, the concept may be personally confronting. But consider this: rigid paralysis is an unequivocal consequence of brain damage whereas relaxation of the musculoskeletal system is the opposite of rigid paralysis. Ideal neurological functioning is illustrated when postures and movements appear effortless. Michael Jordan stood out among his peers not because he was stronger or faster but because he was more graceful. He could put himself in the right place at the right time, and make it look easy. Dancers, gymnasts, and divers are judged by the grace with which they execute their moves. Grace is a reflection of their ability to relax while moving.

My quest for the elusive experience of coziness was actually a quest for the ability to relax—to relax my body, my brain, and my vigilance. My current ability to experience coziness is a reflection of my neurological recovery, and it is the best demonstration of why all my efforts were worthwhile.

Play

Vladimir Janda, a famous Czech neurologist, was motivated to study neurology because of his personal experience as a polio survivor. I was motivated to study with Dr. Janda because of my personal experience with a neurological injury.

Professor Janda once told me that, "if you want your patients to continue to embrace their rehabilitation program, you must keep introducing new toys as therapy." It is not about toys, it is about creating playfulness to support the process. Balls, balance boards, and exercise equipment are the tools of the physical rehabilitation professional. They are also the tools found in athletic facilities and playgrounds. In a similar manner, card games, board games, and chalk marks on a sidewalk are the games of children and the tools of educators. They are also the tools of rehabilitation professionals. The lines between neurological rehabilitation, athletic achievement, and education are blurry. That is a good thing! The general population has experience with both education and athletic endeavors, but not usually with rehabilitation. Neurological rehabilitation is not that different. A good coach, a good educator, and a good health care provider play to their subjects' strengths while addressing the weaknesses. We learn or relearn the alphabet by singing our ABCs. We learn or relearn motor skills by playing games such as jump rope and soccer. We learn or relearn strategies by playing board games and team sports.

Health care providers, family, the community, and injured individuals often approach brain injury as an enemy, which must be defeated. When the experience is that of an army waging a war, there is little room for gratitude and enrichment. Conversely, the structure of play offers amusement and camaraderie, as well as the opportunity to excel.

I have enjoyed—literally enjoyed—years of rehabilitative efforts, both as a physician and as an individual. The beauty of my profession (chiropractic) is that it emphasizes the enhancement of function, in either the presence or absence of pathology. The focus is not on the diagnosis as much as the ability of the individual to function comfortably and effectively. Applying this philosophy, I encourage my patients to incorporate their rehabilitation efforts into their daily lives. I have a patient who chooses cowboy dancing as a medium for vestibular rehabilitation. I prefer contra dancing myself. Another patient combined her exercises into a dance routine she can perform daily; she would rather dance than do homework—which is how she conceptualizes the exercises I give her. Yet another patient incorporates her therapy into her house cleaning activities. Just living life is rehabilitation. For me that is not a bad thing—I am a learner by nature. Play is the construct that makes learning pleasurable.

Connecting with Community

Neurological rehabilitation is by its nature multidisciplinary. There is no single profession, clinic, or hospital that can fully rehabilitate an individual with a brain injury. In the same way that it takes a village to raise a child, it takes a community to habilitate its citizens, including those of us with neurological loss.

My community offers me a variety of ongoing rehabilitation opportunities—none of them labeled or conceptualized as such. These opportunities allow me to challenge myself, but without devastating consequences. They connect me with my physical body, helping me regain a physical experience of intellectual enjoyment. I had to get used to being consistently last and making repeated mistakes, but when I finally embraced that (although it remains an ongoing lesson in letting go), I had the freedom to play within my community.

For instance, I enjoy orienteering: running around with a map and a compass looking for treasure in the wilderness. Despite my neurological losses, I maintain an intrinsic sense of direction and a notion that I can always find my way home safely. However, the devil is in the details: orienteering mimics real-world demands by requiring a combination of close visual work, attention to detail, understanding of time and space, the ability to shift between two-dimensional representation and three dimensional space, coordinated movement, and strategic planning. Successful orienteering also requires one to admit: I am wrong; I made a mistake; I am not where I think I am; and I must back up to succeed.

This is exactly why orienteering is not a popular sport; it is uncomfortable to admit to being lost or wrong. Fortunately, when I make a mistake on the orienteering course I am usually alone, which is a natural consequence of being off course. Orienteering clubs provide a built-in context for comfortably acknowledging mistakes. Mistakes are called errors and ranked in terms of minutes, as in, "I made a four minute error when I went to the left of the ridge rather than to the right." The orienteering event itself is often followed by lively discussion on strategy and errors. Since there is such a range of participants, from 40 years older to 40 years younger than myself, it is possible that I will still be faster, more accurate, or more persistent than at least one other contestant. After years of being last in almost all events, I find this knowledge comforting.

When I first started orienteering I would register under the name of my pet cat, supported by the logic that cats don't worry about making mistakes or looking foolish so neither should I. This worked well. When the results were published, I did not have to publicly own my poor outcomes. Now, since my errors do not affect me as deeply as they once did, I register under my own name and often choose courses that are above my ability level simply to challenge myself. On occasion I have run (actually walked) the course without a compass as a drill designed to improve my map-reading skills.

I played field hockey in a college where I was undoubtedly one of the worst players on the team. However I was good enough to stay on the team, and I had a skill level that I now envy. Tucson has one field hockey club. Fortunately it is a social club, not a competitive team. We have a state-wide reputation as a drinking club with a hockey problem. On its surface this does not sound like an appropriate rehabilitation opportunity. However, my experience on the team has enriched my personal life and fostered my recovery. We meet weekly, divide into teams randomly, and play for several hours without keeping score. We simply play for the pleasure of playing. Skill levels range from Olympic quality to completely inept while ages range from nowhere-near-old-enough-to-belong-to-a-drinking-club to early fifties. I fall into the categories of early fifties and completely inept, even though I have played for 20 years. I confront my losses of coordination, timing, speed, and organization on a weekly basis but in a relatively safe environment (that being said, I have had a few painful bruises as a direct result of my poor coordination on the field). I confront those same losses every day at work, but the impact on my income and career is so profound that I can't bring the same level of playfulness to my workspace. On the hockey field, I can allow myself to be shattered by my poor performance one moment and then pleased with my success the next. My skill level has improved over the years, and the improved function is paralleled throughout my life. It is just more fun to measure it on the field.

Despite our reputation, we are a socially responsible hockey team. Many of us choose not to consume alcohol based on spiritual faith, personal preference, or simply because we are not old enough to order a drink. The rest of us are mature enough to drive home sober. Our reputation speaks to our ability to play for the fun of playing, without concern for winning, losing, or appearing foolish. This is the art of the rehabilitation partnership between a professional and the person with a brain injury.

The Future

Technological advances have served the brain-injured community well. The internet allows individuals to embrace the broader community for education and support. Sensitive imaging supports appropriate diagnosis. Computer-based rehabilitation programs support recovery. Labor saving devices support quality of life. I rarely dial a phone number; memory phones, quick dial, and redial features have obviated the need. And what about typing? As I compose this article, I am grateful for the voice dictation system that makes each word appear before my eyes. I still cannot type efficiently but, thanks to technology, that no longer limits me. The quality of voice dictation systems has improved dramatically over the past several years—just in time to allow me to be far more productive personally and clinically, with much less effort.

In my clinic, technology has enabled me to switch from documenting patient records on paper charts to electronic charts. Electronic health records are a legal requirement in the United States—all clinics must be compliant by 2014. This legislation has raised justifiable concerns about the costs of implementation, privacy, and the heightened level of accountability for health care providers. I find it amusing that a legal requirement that has caused so much outrage has been liberating for me. I can generate an electronic record with much less effort than a paper record—and of course that electronic record is easier to read than my handwriting.

Remarkably, radical improvements in my personal level of function, and the availability of computer-based labor saving devices, have emerged coincident with a heightening awareness of traumatic brain injury. Advancements in medical imaging technology, the escalating number of U.S. military veterans with head injuries, media attention to concussions in professional athletes, and the tragic shooting of a U.S. congressperson in my own neighborhood have all contributed to a heightened awareness of the personal and public impact of neurological insult. This new awareness will drive research, support services, and promote public understanding. It will facilitate a paradigm that allows physicians and laypersons to accept brain injury, and those who have sustained brain injuries, with greater understanding.

It is a perfect time for me—as a human and as a clinician. I have spent a decade working diligently on the residual impact of my head injury while keeping the injury itself in the closet. My infrequent disclosures were poorly received due to the public misperception that head injury is always synonymous with intellectual inadequacy or emotional instability. This is simply not true.

As a physician I have referred patients to other providers, only to see their signs and symptoms misdiagnosed as malingering, or drug abuse—even in the absence of potential for financial gain, a psychiatric disorder, or an indication of past or current drug use. The tragedy is that this misdiagnosis denies them the validity and services that could support them. I have seen patients lose jobs, spouses, academic scholarships, and sense of worth as a direct result of their undiagnosed or misdiagnosed brain injuries. The irony is that these adverse consequences occurred because the initial injury was so subtle.

There is much to be learned from the experiences and support systems of those with other acquired brain insults. For instance, I have referred a few patients and families to postpolio support groups because these groups offered something brain injury groups did not. Postpolio support groups have been in existence for many years, are well organized, have a substantial presence on the internet, and offer well-researched information about community support services. There are many parallels between the characteristic symptoms of postpolio syndrome (PPS) and traumatic brain injury. Polio is by definition a result of a viral insult to the brain. Fatigue, brain fog, autonomic dysregulation, and centrally mediated pain syndromes are common to both conditions and are historically misunderstood by the medical and lay communities. Unfortunately, fatigue, brain fog, and chronic pain continue to be stigmatized conditions. PPS support groups offer education and validation to all individuals with such symptoms.

PPS support groups emerged as a consequence of the polio epidemics in the 1950s, and their demographic constitution reflects this origin. As the population with polio ages, younger generations will take the lead in providing community support and education for these symptoms. These new leaders may be the survivors of physical brain trauma given the growing number of individuals, such as military personnel and professional athletes, who experience a head injury. The adult children of parents who have lived long enough to begin showing signs of dementia or other progressive neurological loss may also take the lead in community support and education.

I can envision a time when a heightened public awareness of neurological insult will drive legislation, research, and community support services. One can expect a spillover effect where an understanding of brain injury supports an appreciation of a host of progressive neurological conditions, such as Lyme disease, viral insult, and chronic fatigue syndrome.

I expect to see partnerships across disciplines and across support groups in the pursuit of good rehabilitation. We have much to share with each other.

The science of rehabilitation involves an intellectual understanding of potential interventions. The art is the experiential understanding of when, and in what sequence, to employ each intervention, and why. The phrase "if you've seen one brain injury, you've seen one brain injury" speaks to the individual nature of each and implies the need for custom-designed rehabilitation treatment plans. The art of rehabilitation question is, what combination of interventions, in what order and with what frequency, will be most effective for this individual in this situation? My rehabilitation efforts, driven more by coincidence than by strategy, were effective but inefficient. The interventions were appropriate, but I would have been better served by applying them at different times, and in a different sequence. Clinical experience and my own loss have helped me develop the art that I now employ with patients.

PART 2

PULLING TOGETHER RATHER THAN FALLING APART: BRAIN INJURY IN FAMILIES

Elizabeth Kendall

Brain injury is an event that is recalled vividly, yet differently, by each family member depending on where they were at the time, how they heard about the injury, their response when they first saw the injured person, and how they interacted with the rehabilitation system in the subsequent years. For family members, memories are provoked by unexpected stimuli at unexpected times, but the details of the event usually appear with the same intensity as they did on the day. The chapters in this section of the book adopt the important perspective of the family as a system following the onset of brain injury. Each chapter acknowledges the role played by different family members—for instance, siblings and children. They show how long-term impacts might occur for these forgotten family members. They also focus on the systemic features of families that influence the way in which they manage the consequences of brain injury. These are critical chapters because, together, they articulate the reciprocal, cyclical, and dynamic nature of brain injury when it occurs within the context of a family. They highlight the importance of considering the systems within which brain injury occurs rather than simply thinking of it as a condition sustained by just one person.

When I started my PhD in 1989, I wanted to focus entirely on the experience of families so I could understand how they coped successfully following brain injury. My intention was to develop a program that could address the needs of families, an intention inspired by my own family experience of brain injury a decade before. This experience had revealed the complete absence of any family-focused support within the health system at the time. Although my PhD topic changed slightly, my research was the start of an important journey that connected me with many families who had faced and survived the challenges created by brain injury. It also brought me into contact with many families in tremendous pain, people whose worlds had been turned upside down and whose lives would never be the same. The enduring resilience of those families continues to impress me, particularly given the lack of services or supports to assist them.

At the same time, I was enthused by Muriel Lezak's (1988) seminal article in the *Journal of Clinical and Experimental Neuropsychology* titled "Brain Damage is a Family Affair." This article heralded an emerging understanding of the impact brain injury could have on family members. Like many articles published around this time, the focus tended to be on the characteristics of the injured person that caused distress for family members. There was a growing body of articles that documented the high rate of family breakdown following brain injury, most of which focused on the negative impact of brain injury on the ability of a person to sustain social relationships. Any interventions directed toward the family tended to focus on assisting individual members to cope as best they could while they confronted the inevitable crises created by brain injury. The ultimate intent of such interventions was to ensure that they could continue supporting their injured family member. These interventions typically involved counseling or therapy that was delivered independent of the person with brain injury. Thus, these therapeutic processes inadvertently segregated the family, creating an artificial divide between the identified problem (whether this be the person with brain injury or the person who was not coping) and the family unit as a whole.

Now, nearly a quarter of a century later, we are finally seeing a real shift in thinking about the role of family in rehabilitation and recovery. Although not fully articulated into practice yet, there is now considerable rhetoric about engaging families as partners in the decision-making process. There is more recognition than ever that family-centered approaches are necessary in rehabilitation. Although still somewhat behind other areas, brain injury systems are beginning to recognize the fact that families can be experts about what works for them, that they are critical to the overall system of care and mutual support and that they are, often, the only constant in an ever-changing service system (Bamm & Rosenbaum, 2008).

In my own research on coping and adjustment conducted since 1990, I have repeatedly found that family functioning at the time of injury was a long-term direct predictor of successful outcome (see Kendall & Terry, 2009). This conclusion was not, however, something I needed 20 years of research to tell me. I experienced brain injury first hand when my brother was injured in a motor vehicle accident 30 years ago. Hit head on by a drunk driver at high speed, he was lucky to have survived. At that time, there was little in the way of rehabilitation where we lived. What little rehabilitation he was offered was not particularly appealing to my brother, who wanted nothing more than to come home from hospital. In response to his obvious distress, his treating physician signed an early discharge, stating that my brother would be far better off at home with his family. The physician told us not to expect too much improvement if we took him home, making it clear that we had no role to play in rehabilitation.

Although it was a difficult time for my family, there never seemed to be any major upheaval. Of course, my brother might have a slightly different interpretation of this time, but as a family, we just continued. I do recall many of the feelings described by the siblings in this section of the book, which naturally led me to seek attention in other, sometimes destructive, ways. But it was not until I began working in the field of brain injury rehabilitation that I realized how lucky we were to have been a relatively stable and well-resourced family for whom brain injury did not create utter devastation. Was ours an example of family resilience as described in this section of the book? I assume it was, although we never thought about it that way. Does it mean we did everything right? Did we provide the right types of support in the right situations as described in this book? I am sure we did not, but we did survive and we might actually have thrived. There is no doubt, though, that it would have been easier with guidance such as that provided in this book.

At the time, the prevailing model in brain injury was one of biomedical intervention, with little credence being given to the role of the family in rehabilitation. Whatever families did to support their relatives, they did by drawing on instinct, understanding, and dedication. In 2005, I read an important piece of research that finally articulated the reason why families should be engaged in rehabilitation. This research compared standard clinician-delivered rehabilitation with a family-supported intervention. It confirmed much of what we had been finding in our own research, but did so in a nicely designed randomized controlled clinical trial (Braga, DaPaz, & Ylvisaker, 2005). The researchers trained parents to deliver rehabilitation to their injured children, thus producing a group of parents who could competently engage their children in therapeutic activities within the routines of daily life in the home. Importantly, the ability to learn these techniques was not associated with the parents' education level or literacy, which is often raised as semilegitimate reasons for not engaging families in rehabilitation. Even more importantly, children in the family-supported group actually demonstrated superior cognitive and physical functioning following one year of treatment.

For many decades, families have been an underutilized resource. They have often been crying out to know how they could engage in and support the rehabilitation of their relatives. Thanks to this important research and other similar work, it is now widely recommended that family members be engaged in the process of rehabilitation. No doubt, barriers will continue to exist from both perspectives—some practitioners will always favor their own dominance, some families will lack the functional capacity or willingness to engage. A major question for the service system is how to ensure that optimal engagement and support is possible for all types of families, regardless of their capacity and in line with their preferences. In cases where families are not able to be engaged for some reason, how can we establish something equivalent in a person's life?

Most importantly, in an age where families are expected to engage in rehabilitation, how can we effectively monitor their well-being to ensure that engagement does not exacerbate the pressure families already experience? Brain injury is a unique dilemma for most families, probably the most challenging many will face in their lifetime. Not only are they confronting the loss of a loved one, at least in a familiar form, but they are simultaneously carrying the weight of being the most important source of support for their relative. How can we support families to juggle this approach-avoidance conflict? On the one hand, they want nothing more than to be helpful and participate in the recovery of their loved one, but on the other hand, they are frustrated, grief-stricken, personally damaged, and frequently bearing the brunt of the injured person's anger. Sometimes, all they want is to get away from the situation, or express their own anger. We should not pretend that it will be easy to help someone else manage such an unresolvable dilemma.

For some family members, the post–brain injury world becomes one of "if only. . ." Nothing will ever alter the fact that their entire family permanently changed on the day of the injury. The influence of brain injury on the family can be profound and pervasive. Over time, it becomes impossible to think about how the family might have been had the injury not occurred. It becomes especially difficult to know what has actually changed as a result of the injury and what might have been the case anyway, especially when the injury has affected a young person or a new family. In thinking about how to help families, I am reminded of a quote from Heinz Kohut, a famous psychotherapist. Kohut said, "The key to therapeutic change may not be insight or understanding, but rather being understood." The chapters in this section of the book have demonstrated that there is clearly a need for better understanding about the experiences of families and the ways in which we can facilitate resilience. If our aim is to improve rehabilitation, then a natural corollary is that we need to understand the families within which rehabilitation occurs.

References

Bamm, E. L., & Rosenbaum, P. (2008). Family-centered theory: Origins, development, Barriers, and supports to implementation in rehabilitation medicine. *Archives of Physical Medicine and Rehabilitation, 89*(8), 1618–1624.

Braga, L. W., da Paz Junior, A. C., & Ylvisaker, M. (2005). Direct clinician-delivered versus indirect family-supported rehabilitation of children with traumatic brain injury: A randomized controlled trial. *Brain Injury, 19*(10), 819–831.

Kendall, E., & Terry, D. (2009). Predicting emotional well-being following traumatic brain injury: A test of mediated and moderated models. *Social Science & Medicine, 69*(6), 947–954.

Lezak, M. D. (1988). Brain damage is a family affair. *Journal of Clinical and Experimental Neuropsychology, 10*(1), 111–123.

IN THEORY

In general theory you should take care of me, patience is for you to
   grant me. That I without you would have no clue.
That is true.
Because I love you, so I depend on you. I need you beyond the routine my body needs. Deeper than the deepest sea into the soul of a
   dreamer that thrives on serendipity. I need you beyond the labels,
   appointments, answers, and all the things that seem so impossi-
   bly easy, yet not for me.
In theory I need you because I can't do this on my own, that it's not
   all. I need you because I love you and embody you. In theory
   it's all logic that pulls, ties us, but reality of heart outlines other
   things that draw me to your side.
True, beyond the twists of shoelaces and zipping of my jacket, my
   awareness feels you there; your love sweetens the air. That is how
   I can do the things I do.
Theories stand so fixed that I mix the logic of life into my reason
   and rhyme.
My theory is you feel the same. You do all the little things, to guide
   me to the feeling that's too big for material space.
Fated by God to not witness but endure what it takes to live in love,
That is my theory.

Erica Anderson

CHAPTER 4

Family Resilience and Traumatic Brain Injury

Michelle McIntyre and Elizabeth Kendall

Resilience, the process of positive adaptation in the face of significant adversity (Luthar, Cicchetti, & Becker, 2000), is an important attribute for families faced with traumatic brain injury (TBI). Not surprisingly, many families struggle to adapt to the significant life changes TBI brings. However, some families demonstrate resilience and positive outcomes after TBI, a fact that has been underreported in the literature (Kendall & Terry, 2008; Machamer, Temkin, & Dikmen, 2002). Family resilience is poorly defined and underresearched in relation to TBI due to an emphasis on negative impacts and outcomes. Consequently, little is known about "positive emotions, resilience, or instances when depression does not occur" (Bowen, Yeates, & Palmer, 2010, p. 285). It is important to note that the resilience paradigm does not seek to minimize the impact of adversity, nor suggest that events such as TBI are anything but extremely challenging for families. The intention is to understand the factors that enable some families to bounce forward (Walsh, 2012) in the face of adversity, weaving meaning and growth into their new realities.

The Importance of Family for People with Traumatic Brain Injury

Understandings of the meaning of "family" have broadened over time to increasingly recognize family diversity and pluralism (Holstein & Gubrium, 1999). In this context family refers to the inner circles of support that mobilize around the injured person, and may include parents, siblings, children, spouse, or significant others. When an individual sustains a TBI, the family typically represents the most significant form of emotional, social, and financial support (Gan & Schuller, 2002). Indeed, research has long indicated an increasing reliance on family, rather than friends, for social support over time (Kozloff, 1987; Oddy, Coughlan, Tyerman, & Jenkins, 1985). Many families also take on responsibility for the long-term care of their injured loved one. Families are an essential part of the rehabilitation process, with family involvement being shown to improve outcomes for the injured person (Braga, da Paz Junior, & Ylvisaker, 2005; Frain et. al., 2007). However, family relationships are prone to deterioration following TBI. For example, high levels of friction have been found in relationships between people with TBI and their parents. Marital relationships have been shown to be more negatively impacted than those of parents and children (Gervasio & Kreutzer, 1997), with marriages frequently ending in divorce (Parente, DiCesare, & Parente, 1990). Spouses report dissatisfaction with the role of carer, perhaps due to the incompatibility of this role with that of sexual partner (Bowen et al., 2009). The perception in adult siblings of people with TBI that the injury resulted in restrictions to family activities and reduced access to social support was found to be correlated with higher levels of sibling depression (Degeneffe & Lynch, 2006). This friction in family relationships following TBI can result in distress and illness for family members, inhibiting relatives' capacity and/or willingness to support the injured person. Indeed, research has indicated that the distress resulting from TBI was as great or greater for family members as for the injured person (Brooks, 1991; Gan & Schuller, 2002; Kosciulek & Lustig, 1998). Family adaptation to the changes associated with TBI is complex, presenting some unique challenges as families renegotiate roles and relationships, often with diminished financial and social resources. Unlike stroke or dementia, which primarily affect the elderly, the prevalence of TBI in young adult males means affected families are usually in the early stages of their development and less equipped to cope (Cavallo & Kay, 2011; Moore, Stambrook, & Peters, 1993).

TBI presents a sudden disruption in continuity, which can have a profound impact on the families' ability to adjust (Cavallo & Kay, 2011). Personality and behavior changes often associated with TBI have been found to cause considerable distress in families (Allen, Linn, Gutierrez, & Willer, 1994; Kreutzer, Gervasio, & Camplair, 1994b), with many reporting a sense that their loved one has become a stranger (Mauss-Clum & Ryan, 1981; Serio, Kreutzer, & Gervasio, 1995). The permanence of the changes and the unpredictability of the injured person's behavior are also contributors to poor long-term family functioning. It is these behavioral problems often associated with TBI that have been shown to have the greatest impact on caregiver and family functioning (Anderson, Parmenter, & Mok, 2002; Ponsford & Schönberger, 2010).

In the face of these challenges, many families struggle to adapt to the impacts of TBI on the family system, resulting in fractured relationships and diminished capacity for long-term family involvement in rehabilitation and care. This crisis within the family system results in increased pressure on services when families are no longer confident about their ability to support a head-injured family member. Understanding the family response to TBI is therefore crucial, as is the provision of appropriate supports for families.

Understanding Families following Traumatic Brain Injury

The last 30 years have seen vast body of research involving families and TBI. Broadly, this research has focused on the impacts and outcomes of TBI for families, the process of family adjustment and adaptation, and the effects of this adaptation on family functioning. This focus represents a shift from an earlier emphasis on individual impacts, to a family system approach that examined changes in family roles and relationships (Dell Orto & Power, 2000; Kay & Cavallo, 1991).

Much of the early research investigated the subjective burden and psychological distress experienced by relatives and carers of persons who sustained TBI. Notable was the work generated by Brooks, Livingston, McKinlay, and colleagues (the Glasgow group). These studies examined injury severity, the impact of neurobehavioral symptoms, and stress and depression in family members. A number of studies concluded that the most significant burden for families derived from emotional, behavioral, and personality changes in the injured person, rather than cognitive or physical disabilities (Brooks, Campsie, Symington, Beattie, & McKinlay, 1986, 1987; McKinlay, Brooks, Bond, Martinage, & Marshall, 1981; Oddy, Humphrey, & Uttley, 1978; Thomsen, 1974). It is these neurobehavioral symptoms such as impulsivity, disinhibition, anger outbursts, and social insensitivity (Cavallo & Kay, 2011) rather than the severity of the injury that were associated with the greatest perceived burden (McKinlay et al., 1981; Oddy et al., 1978), the impacts of which were found to increase over time (Brooks, et al., 1986; Brooks & McKinlay, 1983). Similarly, other studies concluded that, in the long term, character changes in the injured person were the greatest cause of stress for families (Lezak, 1978; Mauss-Clum & Ryan, 1981).

Primary caregivers (usually women) have been shown to experience greater stress than noncarer relatives (Perlesz, Kinsella, & Crowe, 2000), often reporting social isolation, and concomitant anxiety and depression (Mauss-Clum & Ryan, 1981). For men, who are more likely to be secondary or tertiary carers, distress is more commonly reported in terms of anger and fatigue (Perlesz et al., 2000). Adjustment tends to be most difficult for spouses (Kreutzer et al., 1994b; Serio et al., 1995). Comparing the experiences of parents and spouses of people with a TBI, Allen et al. (1994) found parents to be more concerned for their loved one's future, whereas spouses reported more negative emotional responses. Wives of men with TBI were more depressed than wives of men with spinal cord injuries (Rosenbaum & Najenson, 1976).

In contrast to these early studies that were predominantly based on the reports of individual family members, family system studies included the entire family unit as the focus of analysis. The family system perspective recognized the interdependencies between family members and how changes in one member of the system effect the functioning of the entire system (Gan, Campbell, Gemeinhardt, & McFadden, 2006). Family systems theory involves consideration of family dynamics, the structure of the family unit, communication patterns, roles, boundaries, and power relationships (Rothbaum, Rosen, Ujiie, & Uchida, 2002), all of which influence the way families adapt to change. This approach acknowledges the reciprocal interactions between the injured person and the families' capacity to function, underscoring the need for rehabilitation services to support the family as a unit (Larøi, 2003; Maitz & Sachs, 1995; Rolland, 2012).

A number of family system studies have indicated increased rates of unhealthy family functioning after TBI (Anderson, et al., 2002; Ergh, Rapport, Coleman, & Hanks, 2002; Gan & Schuller, 2002; Testa, Malec, Moessner, & Brown, 2006). A range of factors that predict poor family functioning have been identified including behavior changes in the injured person (Kreutzer, Gervasio, & Camplair, 1994a; Ponsford, Olver, Ponsford, & Nelms, 2003; Schönberger, Ponsford, Olver, & Ponsford, 2010), cognitive issues (Ergh, et al., 2002; Machamer, et al., 2002), and the injured person's level of integration into the community (Winstanley, Simpson, Tate, & Myles, 2006). The importance of social support as a buffer for some of the negative impacts of TBI on the family system has also been highlighted (Ergh et al., 2002).

Various family system models have been used to understand the family response to TBI. The family life cycle model (Carter & McGoldrick, 1989) provided the framework for Moore et al. (1993), who categorized stresses on family systems in terms of their source and impacts on family members. The model identified centripetal factors (including measures of family coping, marital adjustment, and number of years married) that held families together, whereas centrifugal factors (number of children, age of oldest child, amount of perceived financial strain) loosened familial bonds. Results highlighted the unique challenges faced by younger developing families when the husband sustained a TBI, particularly when there were financial pressures.

Kosciulek (1996) used Olson's (1993) circumplex model of marital and family systems as a framework for investigating family types. The circumplex model demonstrates the changes families go through at times of crisis in terms of levels of family cohesion (emotional bonding) and adaptability (the ability to change power structure, roles, and relationship rules), which are facilitated by positive communication (Olson, 1993, 2000). Consistent with the model, more balanced families displayed higher levels of positive communication, which facilitated greater flexibility and ability to adapt.

Carnes and Quinn (2005) investigated family adaptation to the role of caregiver, using the Family Adjustment and Adaptation Response (FAAR) model (McCubbin & Patterson, 1983). The FAAR model assessed families from the perspective of stress and coping, and emphasized the four central constructs of *family demands*, balanced with *family capabilities*, which interact with *family meanings*, leading to *family adjustment* or *adaptation* (Patterson, 2002a). Variables found to influence family adaptation included social support, increased financial resources, coping skills, and reframing, and those that added to distress included emotional and behavioral changes in the injured person, and concerns regarding insurance.

Kosciulek and Lustig (1998) applied the Resiliency Model of Family Stress, Adjustment and Adaptation (McCubbin, Thompson, & McCubbin, 1991) to assessment of the relationship between TBI-related family stress and family adaptation. Stressors were identified as follows (Kosciulek & Lustig, 1998, p. 9):

(a) The brain injury and related hardships over time
(b) Normative family cycle transitions such as graduations and marriages
(c) Prior strains accumulated over time
(d) Situational demands and contextual difficulties such as the transition to service systems
(e) Consequences of family efforts to cope such as the handling of anger and grieving
(f) Intrafamily and social ambiguity such as the lack of understanding by friends and disruptions to the family structure

The study concluded that persistent emotional and behavioral problems in the person with the TBI were a major stressor for families and predicted poor family functioning. The pile-up of stressors on families was significant. Positive family adaptation was seen as the process of rebalancing within the family system allowing for organization and unity, and promoting growth and development (Kosciulek & Lustig, 1998).

Dell Orto and Power (2000) summarized the determinants of positive family reaction to brain injury as including previous family history; the meaning ascribed by the family to the injury; family dynamics; coping resources; family status and role of the injured person; the family life cycle stage; the nature of preinjury relationships; available support; cultural background; issues of blame and guilt; and the nature of stressors. Rolland (2012) posited that for families to successfully adapt to sudden onset changes (such as TBI) they must be highly adaptable, cohesive, adept at problem-solving, and capable of reallocating family roles. Despite this volume of theoretical and empirical work, the processes and circumstances involved in positive family adaptation to TBI remain unclear. Understanding family resilience is the necessary and logical next step for family TBI research.

Defining Family Resilience

Early resilience research focused primarily on individual resilience and was typically associated with childhood trauma (Coyle et al., 2009; Patterson, 2002b). The terms resilience and resiliency are grammatically interchangeable. Resilience is used more frequently than resiliency, particularly outside North America. However, some researchers have made a distinction between the stable internal quality of resiliency and more situation-specific resilience. In this chapter, resilience has been used consistently, even when researchers have used the term resiliency. Resilience has increasingly been conceptualized at the family system level, which recognizes the role of the family unit in buffering stress and responding to challenges. This interest in family resilience emerged as a result of changing foci within the two distinct, but related, fields of family studies and psychology, to more positive outcomes and experiences (Patterson, 2002a). This change is evidenced in the moves to strengths-based rather than deficit-based models of family dynamics (Patterson, 2002a), and positive psychology (Seligman & Csikszentmihalyi, 2000). It is reflective of Antonovsky's notion of *salutogenesis* (Antonovsky, 1987), which emphasizes wellness over pathology and asks the question, "what underlies the movement towards health?" (Antonovsky, 1998, p. 7).

There is no single agreed-upon definition of resilience. Resilience has been defined as "the human ability to adapt in the face of tragedy, trauma, adversity, hardship and ongoing significant life stressors" (Newman, 2005, p. 227). McCubbin and colleagues' development of the Resiliency Model was the first time the notion of resilience had been applied to family adaptation (McCubbin & McCubbin, 1988, 1993; McCubbin et al., 1991). This model considered resilience at the family system level, rather than at the individual level and attempted to explain why some families recovered while others deteriorated under the same circumstances (McCubbin, Thompson, & McCubbin, 1996). Central to the model is the notion that family stress can be predictive of family adaptation, with stress referring to the accumulated demands endured by the family system following a major crisis (McCubbin et al., 1991). Factors such as the type of family (regenerative, resilient, rhythmic), family resources, the level of vulnerability, coping and problem-solving capacity, and the family's appraisal of the event were seen to be predictive of the level of adaptation to stressors (Hawley, 2000). The family schema, or world view, was also seen to impact on resilience. Families who perceived life events as comprehensible, manageable, and meaningful were seen to possess a *sense of coherence* (Antonovsky, 1987, 1998), which was associated with positive adaptation. The family adaptation research attempted to determine why some families were able to cope better than others after a crisis. Within the McCubbin model, resiliency is defined as, "the positive behavioral patterns and functional competence individuals and the family unit demonstrate under stressful or adverse circumstances, which determine the family's ability to recover by maintaining its integrity as a family unit" (McCubbin, et al., 1996, p. 5). Here, resilience was conceptualized as a regaining of equilibrium, or a return to pretrauma functioning. Walsh (2003, 2012) extended notions of family resilience to encompass those qualities that arise to combat adversity, moving from resilience as a process of *managing* adversity to one of *transcending* adversity. Beyond endurance and coping, family systems are seen to be strengthened by resources that arise in response to challenges (Rolland & Walsh, 2006). Family resilience is seen not as a fixed set of qualities, but as an emergent process over time, which is affected by biopsychosocial and developmental influences, and is unique to each family (Hawley, 2000; Walsh, 2012). The key processes of family resilience described by Walsh included belief systems (the families' appraisal of the event, including meaning-making, positive outlook, and transcendence or spirituality); organizational patterns (including flexibility, connectedness/cohesion; social and economic resources); and communication/problem-solving (including clarity, emotional expression and collaborative problem-solving) (Walsh, 2012).

Apart from a few exceptions there are scant examples of research investigating family resilience in relation to TBI (Kosciulek & Lustig, 1998; Kosciulek, McCubbin, & McCubbin, 1993; Rees, 2011). A small number of researchers have long noted this dearth of research investigating the process of resilience in families following TBI, and how positive changes in these families have been largely overlooked (Adams, 1996; Perlesz, Kinsella & Crowe, 1999; Ridley, 1989). An overemphasis on family crisis and negative functioning means that understandings of healthy family adaptation remain elusive (Rolland, 2012). Existing research has provided invaluable insights into the challenges facing people with TBI and their families, but there are significant gaps in knowledge about families who recover, repair, and grow through adversity. It has been found that families do report some positive changes after TBI. For instance, in one study investigating significant other burden, 60 percent reported their overall experience as being more positive than negative, and 93 percent were reportedly happy to care for their loved one (Machamer et al., 2002). Similarly, a study conducted by Knight, Devereux, and Godfrey (1998) revealed that many of the negative reports from primary caregivers were balanced by comments expressing resolve in the face of adversity, improvements in spousal relationships, and descriptions of caregiving as being uplifting. However these examples are the exception, and positive findings have usually emerged from research focused on other facets of TBI. Studies explicitly focused on family strengths and positive experiences are rare. A comprehensive understanding of the processes of family resilience after TBI is needed to illuminate the path to appropriate interventions.

Family Resilience and Clinical Practice

It has been noted that although there is an abundance of research highlighting the profound effect TBI has on families, there is inadequate support available for families (Frain et al., 2007), and very little evidence for effective family interventions (Boschen, Gargaro, Gan, Gerber, & Brandys, 2007; Bowen et al., 2010; Foster et al., 2012). A review of family interventions in this area identified seven categories of interventions: educational interventions; telephone/internet-delivered support; case management; counseling; support group/peer support; and multicomponent interventions (Boschen et al., 2007). There was a tendency for interventions to be aimed at the individual, indicating a failure to acknowledge that those designed to support the entire family unit are more likely to be effective than those targeting individual members (Gan et al., 2006). A family system approach was evident in one study (Charles, Butera-Prinzi, & Perlesz, 2007), which used family group work. Although family dysfunction continued, parents' personal distress levels were reduced, and families reported benefits such as a greater understanding of brain injury, mutual support and sharing, lessened feelings of shame and social isolation, and shifts from feelings of blame to compassion.

Interventions designed to build family resilience acknowledge the importance of the family system, and the latent potential of this system to recover and heal after trauma. A resilience approach entails a shift in focus from areas of deficiency to an assessment of family challenges, "with the conviction in the potential inherent in family systems for recovery and positive growth out of adversity" (Walsh, 2012, p. 422). Applying a resilience framework to family interventions involves collaboration, with the aim of harnessing internal and external family resources. This implies reflexive, flexible approaches, tailored to the unique characteristics of each family system.

Hawley (2000) noted the diverse and dynamic character of family resilience, suggesting the need for recognition of resilience as a developmental pathway, a need to identify commonalities among varying resilience pathways, and a focus on assisting families to identify and develop a useful family schema. Focusing on family strengths has been repeatedly stressed as a key strategy for supporting positive family functioning and resilience (Hawley, 2000; Walsh, 2012; Ylvén, Björck-Åkesson, & Granlund, 2006). The importance of families developing an understanding of their strengths and the ways in which they function positively was further emphasized by Rolland (2012). The families' capacity to make meaning of their experiences and to possess a sense that they are capable of managing adversity is crucial to family resilience (Rolland, 2012).

According to Walsh (2012), interventions that aim to strengthen the key processes for resilience will promote family resources. Approaches that build family resilience offer promise and have the potential to provide much needed support for families after TBI. However, more research is needed in this area to suggest effective strategies for implementing such an approach within our existing health and rehabilitation systems. Continuing to focus on individuals rather than family units means that we are overlooking one of the greatest sources of support for people with TBI. Family is clearly meaningful, and supporting family resilience is a crucial investment for the future.

References

Adams, N. (1996). Positive outcomes in families following traumatic brain injury (TBI). *Australian and New Zealand Journal of Family Therapy, 17*(2), 75–84.

Allen, K., Linn, R. T., Gutierrez, H., & Willer, B. S. (1994). Family burden following traumatic brain injury. *Rehabilitation Psychology, 39*(1), 29–48.

Anderson, M. I., Parmenter, T. R., & Mok, M. (2002). The relationship between neurobehavioural problems of severe traumatic brain injury (TBI), family functioning and the psychological well-being of the spouse/caregiver: path model analysis. *Brain Injury, 16*(9), 743–757.

Antonovsky, A. (1987). *Unraveling the mystery of health*. San Francisco: Jossey-Bass.

Antonovsky, A. (1998). The sense of coherence. An historical and future perspective. In H. I. McCubbin, E. A. Thompson, A. I. Thompson, & J. E. Fromer (Eds.), *Stress, coping, and health in families: sense of coherence and resiliency* (pp. 3–20). Thousand Oaks, CA: Sage.

Boschen, K., Gargaro, J., Gan, C., Gerber, G., & Brandys, C. (2007). Family interventions after acquired brain injury and other chronic conditions: a critical appraisal of the quality of the evidence. *Neurorehabilitation, 22*(1), 19–41.

Bowen, C., Hall, T., Newby, G., Walsh, B., Weatherhead, S., & Yeates, G. (2009). The impact of brain injury on relationships across the lifespan and across school, family and work contexts. *Human Systems, 20*(1), 65–80.

Bowen, C., Yeates, G., & Palmer, S. (2010). *A relational approach to rehabilitation: Thinking about relationships after brain injury*. London: Karnac Books.

Braga, L. W., da Paz Junior, A. C., & Ylvisaker, M. (2005). Direct clinician-delivered versus indirect family-supported rehabilitation of children with traumatic brain injury: a randomized controlled trial. *Brain Injury, 19*(10), 819–831Brooks, N. (1991). The head injured family. *Journal of Clinical and Experimental Neuropsychology, 13*(1), 155–188.

Brooks, N., Campsie, L., Symington, C., Beattie, A., & McKinlay, W. (1986). The five year outcome of severe blunt head injury: a relative's view. *Journal of Neurology, Neurosurgery, and Psychiatry, 49*(7), 764–770.

Brooks, N., Campsie, L., Symington, C., Beattie, A., & McKinlay, W. (1987). The effects of severe head injury on patient and relative within seven years of injury. *Journal of Head Trauma Rehabilitation, 2*(3), 1–13.

Brooks, N., & McKinlay, W. (1983). Personality and behavioural change after severe blunt head injury—a relative's view. *Journal of Neurology, Neurosurgery, and Psychiatry, 46*(4), 336–344.

Carnes, S. L., & Quinn, W. H. (2005). Family adaptation to brain injury: Coping and psychological distress. *Families, Systems, & Health, 23*(2), 186–203.

Carter, E., & McGoldrick, M. (Eds.). (1989). *The changing family life cycle: a framework for family therapy* (2nd ed.). Boston: Allyn and Bacon.

Cavallo, M. M., & Kay, T. (2011). The family system. In J. Silver, T. W. McAllister, & S. C. Yudofsky (Eds.), *Textbook of traumatic brain injury* (2nd ed., pp. 483–504). Washington, D.C.: American Psychiatric Pub.

Charles, N., Butera-Prinzi, F., & Perlesz, A. (2007). Families living with acquired brain injury: a multiple family group experience. *Neurorehabilitation, 22*(1), 61–76.

Coyle, J. P., Macdonald, S., Maguin, E., Safyer, A., DeWit, D., & Nochajski, T. (2009). An exploratory study of the nature of family resilience in families affected by parental alcohol abuse. *Journal of Family Issues, 30*(12), 1606–1623.

Degeneffe, C. E., & Lynch, R. T. (2006). Correlates of depression in adult siblings of persons with traumatic brain injury. *Rehabilitation Counseling Bulletin, 49*(3), 130–142.

Dell Orto, A. E., & Power, P. W. (2000). *Brain injury and the family: a life and living perspective*. Boca Raton, FL: CRC Press.

Ergh, T. C., Rapport, L. J., Coleman, R. D., & Hanks, R. A. (2002). Predictors of caregiver and family functioning following traumatic brain injury: social support moderates caregiver distress. *The Journal of Head Trauma Rehabilitation, 17*(2), 155–174.

Foster, A. M., Armstrong, J., Buckley, A., Sherry, J., Young, T., Folaki, S., TeMiria, J.H., Theadom, A. & McPherson, K. M. (2012). Encouraging family engagement in the rehabilitation process: a rehabilitation provider's development of support strategies for family members of people with traumatic brain injury. *Disability and rehabilitation, 34*(22), 1855-1862.

Frain, M. P., Berven, N. L., Tschopp, M. K., Lee, G. K., Tansey, T., & Chronister, J. (2007). Use of the resiliency model of family stress, adjustment and adaptation by rehabilitation counselors. *Journal of Rehabilitation, 73*(3), 18–25.

Gan, C., Campbell, K. A., Gemeinhardt, M., & McFadden, G. T. (2006). Predictors of family system functioning after brain injury. *Brain Injury, 20*(6), 587–600.

Gan, C., & Schuller, R. (2002). Family system outcome following acquired brain injury: clinical and research perspectives. *Brain Injury, 16*(4), 311–322.

Gervasio, A. H., & Kreutzer, J. S. (1997). Kinship and family members' psychological distress after traumatic brain injury: a large sample study. *Journal of Head Trauma Rehabilitation, 12*(3), 14–26.

Hawley, D. R. (2000). Clinical implications of family resilience. *American Journal of Family Therapy, 28*(2), 101–116.

Holstein, J. A., & Gubrium, J. (1999). What is family? *Marriage & Family Review, 28*(3–4), 3–20.

Kay, T., & Cavallo, M. M. (1991). Evolutions: research and clinical perspectives on families. In J. M. Williams & T. Kay (Eds.), *Head injury: a family matter* (pp. 121–150). Baltimore: Paul H. Brookes.

Kendall, E., & Terry, D. J. (2008). Understanding adjustment following traumatic brain injury: is the goodness-of-fit coping hypothesis useful? *Social Science & Medicine, 67*(8), 1217–1224.

Knight, R. G., Devereux, R., & Godfrey, H. P. (1998). Caring for a family member with a traumatic brain injury. [Research Support, Non-U.S. Govt]. *Brain Injury, 12*(6), 467–481.

Kosciulek, J. F. (1996). The circumplex model and head injury family types: a test of the balanced versus extreme hypotheses. *Journal of Rehabilitation, 62*(2), 49–54.

Kosciulek, J. F., McCubbin, H. I., & McCubbin, M. A. (1993). A theoretical framework for family adaptation to head-injury. *Journal of Rehabilitation, 59*(3), 40–45.

Kosciulek, J. F., & Lustig, D.C. (1998). Predicting family adaptation from brain injury-related family stress. *Journal of Applied Rehabilitation Counseling, 29*(1), 8–12.

Kozloff, R. (1987). Networks of social support and the outcome from severe head injury. *Journal of Head Trauma Rehabilitation, 2*(3), 14–23.

Kreutzer, J. S., Gervasio, A. H., & Camplair, P. S. (1994a). Patient correlates of caregivers' distress and family functioning after traumatic brain injury. *Brain Injury, 8*(3), 211–230.

Kreutzer, J. S., Gervasio, A. H., & Camplair, P. S. (1994b). Primary caregivers' psychological status and family functioning after traumatic brain injury. *Brain Injury, 8*(3), 197–210.

Larøi, F. (2003). The family systems approach to treating families of persons with brain injury: a potential collaboration between family therapist and brain injury professional. *Brain Injury, 17*(2), 175–187.

Lezak, M. D. (1978). Living with the characterologically brain injured patient. *Journal of Clinical Psychiatry, 39*(7), 592–598.

Luthar, S. S., Cicchetti, D., & Becker, B. (2000). The construct of resilience: a critical evaluation and guidelines for future work. *Child Development, 71*(3), 543–562.

Machamer, J., Temkin, N., & Dikmen, S. (2002). Significant other burden and factors related to it in traumatic brain injury. *Journal of Clinical and Experimental Neuropsychology, 24*(4), 420–433.

Maitz, E. A., & Sachs, P. R. (1995). Treating families of individuals with traumatic brain injury from a family system's perspective. *Journal of Head Trauma Rehabilitation, 10*(2), 1–11

Mauss-Clum, N., & Ryan, M. (1981). Brain injury and the family. *Journal of Neuroscience Nursing, 13*(4), 165–169.

McCubbin, H. I., & McCubbin, M. A. (1988). Typologies of resilient families: Emerging roles of social class and ethnicity. *Family Relations, 37*(3), 247–254.

McCubbin, H. I., & McCubbin, M. A. (1993). Family coping with health crises: the resiliency model of family stress, adjustment, and adaptation. In C. B. Danielson, B. Hamel-Bissell, & P. Winstead-Fry (Eds.), *Families, health & illness: perspectives on coping and intervention.* St. Louis: Mosby.

McCubbin, H. I., & Patterson, J. M. (1983). The family stress process: The double ABC-X model of adjustment and adaptation. In H. I. McCubbin, M. B. Sussman, & J. M. Patterson (Eds.), *Social stress and the family: Advances and development in family stress theory and research.* (pp. 7–37). Stroud, Gloucestershire: Hawthorne Press.

McCubbin, H. I., Thompson, A. I., & McCubbin, M. A. (1991). Family stress theory and assessment: the resiliency model of family stress, adjustment and adaptation. In H. I. McCubbin, & A. I. Thompson (Eds.), *Family assessment inventories for research and practice.* (pp. 3–32). Madison, WI: Family Stress, Coping and Health Project, University of Wisconsin–Madison.

McCubbin, H. I., Thompson, A. I., & McCubbin, M. A. (1996). *Family assessment: Resiliency, coping and adaptation: Inventories for research and practice.* Madison, WI: University of Wisconsin.

McKinlay, W. W., Brooks, D. N., Bond, M. R., Martinage, D. P., & Marshall, M. M. (1981). The short-term outcome of severe blunt head injury as reported by relatives of the injured persons. *Journal of Neurology, Neurosurgery, and Psychiatry, 44*(6), 527–533.

Moore, A., Stambrook, M., & Peters, L. (1993). Centripetal and centrifugal family life cycle factors in long-term outcome following traumatic brain injury. *Brain Injury, 7*(3), 247–255.

Newman, R. (2005). APA's resilience initiative. *Professional Psychology: Research and Practice, 36*(3), 227–229.

Oddy, M., Coughlan, T., Tyerman, A., & Jenkins, D. (1985). Social adjustment after closed head injury: a further follow-up seven years after injury. *Journal of Neurology, Neurosurgery, and Psychiatry, 48*(6), 564–568.

Oddy, M., Humphrey, M., & Uttley, D. (1978). Stresses upon the relatives of head-injured patients. *The British Journal of Psychiatry: The Journal of Mental Science, 133*(6), 507–513.

Olson, D. H. (1993). Circumplex model of marital and family systems. In F. Walsh (Ed.), *Normal family processes.* New York: Guilford Press.

Olson, D. H. (2000). Circumplex model of marital and family systems. *Journal of Family Therapy, 22*(2), 144–167.

Parente, J., DiCesare, A., & Parente, R. (1990). Spouses who stayed. *Cognitive Rehabilitation, 8*, 22–25.

Patterson, J. M. (2002a). Integrating family resilience and family stress theory. *Journal of Marriage and Family, 64*(2), 349–360.

Patterson, J. M. (2002b). Understanding family resilience. *Journal of Clinical Psychology, 58*(3), 233–246.

Perlesz, A., Kinsella, G., & Crowe, S. (1999). Impact of traumatic brain injury on the family: a critical review. *Rehabilitation Psychology, 44*(1), 6–35.

Perlesz, A., Kinsella, G., & Crowe, S. (2000). Psychological distress and family satisfaction following traumatic brain injury: Injured individuals and their primary, secondary, and tertiary carers. *The Journal of Head Trauma Rehabilitation, 15*(3), 909–929.

Ponsford, J., Olver, J., Ponsford, M., & Nelms, R. (2003). Long-term adjustment of families following traumatic brain injury where comprehensive rehabilitation has been provided. *Brain Injury, 17*(6), 453–468.

Ponsford, J., & Schönberger, M. (2010). Family functioning and emotional state two and five years after traumatic brain injury. *Journal of the International Neuropsychological Society, 16*(2), 306–317.

Rees, R. J. (2011). *Out of calamity: Stories of trauma survivors.* Adelaide: Axiom Australia.

Ridley, B. (1989). Family response in head injury: Denial . . . or hope for the future? *Social Science & Medicine, 29*(4), 555–561.

Rolland, J. S. (2012). Mastering family challenges in serious illness and disability. In F. Walsh (Ed.), *Normal family processes: growing diversity and complexity* (4th ed., pp. 452–482). New York: Guilford Publications, Inc.

Rolland, J. S., & Walsh, F. (2006). Facilitating family resilience with childhood illness and disability. *Current Opinion in Pediatrics, 18*(5), 527–538.

Rosenbaum, M., & Najenson, T. (1976). Changes in life patterns and symptoms of low mood as reported by wives of severely brain-injured soldiers. *Journal of Consulting and Clinical Psychology, 44*(6), 881–888.

Rothbaum, F., Rosen, K., Ujiie, T., & Uchida, N. (2002). Family systems theory, attachment theory, and culture. *Family Process, 41*(3), 328–350.

Schönberger, M., Ponsford, J., Olver, J., & Ponsford, M. (2010). A longitudinal study of family functioning after TBI and relatives' emotional status. *Neuropsychological Rehabilitation, 20*(6), 813–829.

Seligman, M. E. P., & Csikszentmihalyi, M. (2000). Positive psychology: an introduction. *American Psychologist, 55*(1), 5–14.

Serio, C. D., Kreutzer, J. S., & Gervasio, A. H. (1995). Predicting family needs after brain injury—Implications for intervention. *Journal of Head Trauma Rehabilitation, 10*(2), 32–45.

Testa, J. A., Malec, J. F., Moessner, A.M., & Brown, A. W. (2006). Predicting family functioning after TBI: impact of neurobehavioral factors. *The Journal of Head Trauma Rehabilitation, 21*(3), 236–247.

Thomsen, I. V. (1974). The patient with severe head injury and his family: a follow-up study of 50 patients. *Scandinavian Journal of Rehabilitation Medicine, 6*(4), 180–183.

Walsh, F. (2003). Family resilience: a framework for clinical practice. *Family Process, 42*(1), 1–18.

Walsh, F. (2012). Family resilience: strengths forged through adversity. In F. Walsh (Ed.), *Normal family processes: Growing Diversity and Complexity* (4th ed., pp. 399–451). New York: Guilford.

Winstanley, J., Simpson, G., Tate, R., & Myles, B. (2006). Early indicators and contributors to psychological distress in relatives during rehabilitation following severe traumatic brain injury. *Journal of Head Trauma Rehabilitation, 21*(6), 453–466.

Ylvén, R., Björck-Åkesson, E., & Granlund, M. (2006). Literature review of positive functioning in families with children with a disability. *Journal of Policy and Practice in Intellectual Disabilities, 3*(4), 253–270.

CHAPTER 5

Someone to Care: Social Support after Brain Injury

Melissa Kendall

Research suggests that support networks alter considerably in size and structure after acquired brain injury (ABI) (Finset, Dyrnes, Krogstad, & Berstad, 1995). Zencius and Wesolowski (1999) found that people with ABI have significantly smaller networks than their able-bodied counterparts—an average of 7 network members compared to 23 respectively. However, family members and professional staff were more commonly found in ABI support networks compared to able-bodied individuals, with the latter networks consisting mainly of friends and coworkers.

More than two decades ago, Elsass and Kinsella (1987) found that 15 percent of their sample with ABI lacked any friends or acquaintances, relying on family rather than friends for satisfaction of their social needs. At the same time, Kozloff (1987) investigated the changes in social interaction patterns subsequent to ABI. He found that during the first few months after injury, both family and friends offered help and support. After this early phase of recovery, interaction with friends decreased dramatically and individuals became increasingly dependent on primary kin. There was also an increase in the utilization of professionals for support (Willer & Corrigan, 1994). In short, many individuals with ABI are likely to have a depleted social support network that is likely to decrease over time and may result in more demand on families and an increased reliance on professionals.

Current evidence suggests that although the size and structure of social networks are affected by ABI, the quality of the support provided is also important to recovery. Even if an adequate support network is available, it has been found that the quality of social support is often reduced (Glass & Maddox, 1992). Social relationships tend to be qualitatively inferior following ABI and individuals rarely receive support commensurate with their needs. Support may be emotional (addressing emotions), practical (addressing the problem), or information based (addressing perceptions) (McColl, Lei, & Skinner, 1995). Kreutzer, Marwitz, and Kepler (1992) suggested that people with ABI may require increased emotional support, but their social networks are often unwilling or unable to provide this type of support, particularly in an ongoing way. Further, relationships formed following ABI are often transient and lack the level of intimacy that is required to facilitate the provision of emotional support (Kozloff, 1987).

To fully understand the complex nature of social support, we must be able to identify exactly how social support needs vary across the different life situations that people with ABI face on a daily basis. Social support does not occur in a vacuum, but within the context of the personal and environmental demands placed on the individual (Gauvin-Lepage & Lefebvre, 2010). Because different events pose different demands, it stands to reason that different kinds of support might be beneficial in different circumstances (Cutrona & Suhr, 1992). Indeed, Jacobson (1986) proposed that effective social support depended on the match between need and the nature of the actual support received. Different stressful situations create needs for different types and amounts of social support. Therefore, social support must be tailored to suit the needs created by the particular setting and the individual's preferences in that setting. Clearly, given the same objective situation, individuals will vary in their assessment of their needs. Further, Coyne, Ellard, and Smith (1990) proposed that some supposedly supportive interactions may have negative or deleterious effects if applied inappropriately. Although social support must be examined in terms of the match between ideal and actual support, the interaction between the source of the support and the type of support is also important. Indeed, studies have identified differences in perceived usefulness of support depending on the source. For instance, Seeman and Berkman (1988) found that emotional support was perceived to be more helpful if it came from friends whereas practical support was considered to be more appropriate when received from family members.

This chapter explores the perceived social support needs of people with ABI and the ways in which their current support systems are meeting those support needs. It examines the ways in which the personal and environmental contexts of the individual may determine social support need. Vignettes of common life situations experienced following ABI (developed from the literature and focus groups) were used as situational backdrops, and described 16 events that broadly represented the domains of tangible assets (shopping experiences, difficulties with memory, experience of rehabilitation, and financial strain), achievement (acquiring self-esteem, planning and organization, controlling behavior, and lost

Table 5.1 Demographic characteristics of sample (*n* = 15)

Age		Mean = 41.8 yrs (Range = 20–61 yrs, *SD* = 12.8 yrs)
Time since injury		Mean = 8.7 yrs (Range = 18 mths to 19 yrs, *SD* = 5.6 yrs)
Length of unconsciousness		Mean = 17.7 days (Range = 0 to 60 days, *SD* = 18.3 days)
Length of hospital stay		Mean = 7.6 mths (Range = 0 to 66 mths, *SD* = 16.4 mths)
Gender	Male	10 (67%)
	Female	5 (33%)
Marital status pre injury	Married	3 (20%)
	Defacto	4 (27%)
	Single	5 (33%)
	Divorced/separated	3 (20%)
Marital status post injury	Married	4 (27%)
	Defacto	2 (13%)
	Single	6 (40%)
	Divorced/separated	3 (20%)
Current living situation	Parents	1 (7%)
	Partners	6 (40%)
	Children only	2 (13%)
	Group	1 (7%)
	Alone	5 (33%)
Employment pre injury	Professional roles	2 (13%)
	Skilled roles	5 (33%)
	Unskilled roles	3 (20%)
	Student	3 (20%)
	Unemployed	2 (13%)
Current employment	Part time unskilled	2 (13%)
	Student	1 (7%)
	Unemployed	13 (80%)
Cause of injury	Motor vehicle accident	6 (40%)
	Fall	4 (26%)
	Assault	3 (20%)
	Surfing	1 (7%)
	Stroke	1 (7%)
Compensation status	Compensable	6 (40%)
	Non compensable	9 (60%)

opportunities), relationships (withdrawal from others, shyness, loss of a partner, and loss of friends) and roles (role change, loss of identity, recognition from others, and discrimination) that had been identified by Cutrona and Russell (1990). The vignettes were brief to ensure that they did not place demands on memory, and were broad enough to encompass a variety of individual experiences. Fifteen people with ABI were identified through a local community-based consumer organization, ensuring an adequate representation of people at different times since injury. Demographic details are provided in Table 5.1.

The people with ABI were presented with each of the 16 vignettes and asked if they had experienced a similar situation. If they identified with the scenario, they were asked to nominate the type of support they would like to receive in that situation (support needed) and from whom they would like to receive that support (source needed). They were also asked to identify the type of support they had actually received (support received) in that situation and who had provided it (source received). Direct comments made by the people with ABI are enclosed within quotation marks to illustrate the conclusions.

The Nature of Social Networks

Social networks represent the structural framework from which social support emerges and, therefore, an important consideration of any study on social support: "You need structure, like a backbone in the body. . . . You need a social network to get you out of yourself." People with ABI identified social network sizes of between 7 and 76 people. The mean social network size identified was 21 people ($SD = 22.6$). The network consisted of those who could potentially provide support, but when members who did not actually provide support were removed, actual social network size ranged from 2 to 43 with a mean of 10 people ($SD = 10.1$). Therefore, although people with ABI identified a large number of people who could potentially provide support to them, only about half of those network members were considered to be active support providers. Sometimes this was related to geographic separation where large distances separated family or friends: "My family and friends they live in remote areas, different areas . . . they had to learn about me by remote control." Others spoke of separation related to people's investment in their own lives, "everyone's caught up in their own lives and I don't have many friends really." Sometimes individuals just lacked access to people "at first I couldn't even talk . . . I'm now at the stage where I can contribute I think . . . except I meet no people to talk to." Indeed, Lefebvre, Cloutier, and Levert (2008) found that even after 10 years, many people with ABI continued to feel left out, isolated, or cut off from family and friends. These individuals often become isolated early following injury.

Siblings were commonly identified as important network members, although in many instances, they were geographically separated from the individual, a finding replicated in the study conducted by Degeneffe and Lee (2010), for instance, "my brother he understands a lot more than the others, and he's quite supportive, he's easy to talk to." Siblings often shared strong bonds because of their common cultural, genetic, and environmental characteristics and they were potentially the longest of all family relationships (Pruchno, Patrick, & Burant, 1996).

Parents were identified as active supports by only 12 people. In some instances, their involvement in the network was perceived to exist only through obligation: "My family [members] still ring me and come and see me and ask me places, same as what they always have see, 'cause they are blood so they have no choice." Some people perceived their reliance on parents to be inappropriate: "I've got mum and dad but give me a break. Thirty-one [years old] and all I can do is go up to mummy and daddy, you know, please."

Some people identified work-related supports, such as employers and colleagues: "My boss . . . he is a support to me. Always hangs shit on me but treats me like anybody else." Rotondi, Sinkule, Balzer, Harris, and Moldovan (2007) confirmed the importance of employer support. Indeed, work roles were recognized as one way in which friendships with colleagues could be made to enhance social networks: "I got a job in a pub, met some people, my own friends."

A reasonably large number of friends and neighbors were contained in the overall social networks, but this number declined significantly when only the close network was considered. As one person stated, "I don't have much in the way of friends . . . I'd like more friends . . . I don't have any personal friends at all, any close friends." Gauvin-Lepage and Lefebvre (2010), in a study of adolescents, found that professionals often believed that the loss of friends and change in friendship networks was inevitable following ABI. However, some individuals stated that friends they had acquired since their injury were more stable members of their social network: "I have quite a few friends that have been pretty good because they accept me for who I am . . . they only know me now so they just think that this is the way I have always been." Robison et al. (2009) stated that friends needed to be flexible, offer encouragement, and make allowances, which may be more possible for friends who had no knowledge of an individual prior to the injury.

Other individuals with ABI were sometimes recognized as being important members of a social network, but were not usually considered to be friends: "I mean I have been to a group at [ABI support group] and that is OK but, you know, it isn't like I want all my friends to be people with a head injury." Indeed, Struchen and colleagues (2011) found that peer mentoring programs aimed at improving networks resulted in improvements in perceived social support, but no change in social activity level or social network size. There was a sense of kinship that formed among people with ABI: "you feel better among your own, that's how I look at it. We have a better understanding." This was particularly the case where other support systems were failing the individual: "We all ended up being like close friends, we just clung together because we all felt that the system just wasn't there for us."

Societal expectations and limited knowledge of brain injury isolated people in the community, which further decreased their network size. Many expectations were related to the lack of visible disability following ABI:

> I've been trying to explain to my family and other people because you don't have your brain in a wheelchair, you've got no credibility. You haven't got a T-shirt, I don't want to wear a badge . . . People abandon you and they reject you because they don't know how to deal with it.

People often spoke of the importance of public perceptions: "People see what you can't do, not what you can do, even though what you can do may be different to what you used to do." This lack of awareness and understanding amongst others required education: "educating the people who are treating me that way. Giving me a chance to prove that I am or I can do, instead of just saying oh you can't do that, you've got a brain injury." Many people with ABI were not able to provide this education themselves, for example, "people's perception of me. I couldn't change their perception of me at the time, because of the way I was." Research supports the notion that the public generally are either unprepared or unwilling to understand and accept someone who is different (Swift & Wilson, 2001). Importantly, however, in addition to lack of knowledge, families and professionals also often harbor misconceptions about ABI (Paterson & Stewart, 2002).

Interestingly, the number of family members in the social network decreased significantly when considering the close network, which was sometimes related to the aging of parents, "them being elderly, they can't do things." Indeed, Minnes, Woodford, Carlson, Johnston, and McColl (2010) found that aging parents identified concerns about their incapacity to provide for the ongoing needs of the person in relation to emotional and social support, creation of opportunities for them to make friends, and their involvement in the community. Sometimes the lack of close family members was perceived as abandonment: "I have two sons and a daughter. I have 10 brothers and sisters. None of them speak to me since my head injury . . . they don't want to know me . . . that like really hurt from my own family." The lack of closeness of family members was also linked to the behavior of the person toward the family: "There is [sic] only two people that I take it [my general frustration] out on, and they are the people that are very close to me, they are the ones that I let go at."

Some people commented on relationship breakdown "I didn't know about my head injury when I married him. When we found out, he couldn't cope with it and I don't think he really cared . . . didn't want the burden." Rates of separation and divorce have been reported in the literature to range from 15 to 54 percent (Gill, Sander, Robins, Mazzei, & Struchen,

2011). Some people stressed the need for a romantic partner but the difficulty in finding anyone, "at this stage I am trying my hardest to get another half, but it's not as easy as people think." Others developed inappropriate relationships in an attempt to seek needed support, "I got involved with a male nurse that I met in the hospital . . . and I moved in with him and his friends . . . because I'm disabled some of them didn't treat me so nice."

Professionals, when identified, were always included in the close network. Indeed, in some instances, professionals were seen as friends: "well it is their job but I'd be friends with them anyway if I had met them as strangers, because I just find them all so helpful." Doig, Fleming, Cornwell, and Kuipers (2011) found that professionals were often considered to be friends, especially when they met individuals in their own home environments. Similarly, Muenchberger, Sunderland, Kendall, and Quinn (2011) found, in a study of residential facilities, that paid friendships with carers were often valued in the absence of other social opportunities. As one person stated, "I know that they're there. I don't need them but I go back to hospital pretty regularly, meet everyone, keep in touch with them." The absence of natural supports increased the need for professional supports (Tomberg, Toomela, Ennok, & Tikk, 2007).

Sometimes individuals instigated the reduction of their own support networks following ABI as a protection strategy: "I've turned reclusiveness into an art form . . . almost a protection, the less you have to do, the less interaction with people, the more protected you are." In other instances, reduced support networks resulted from the inability of the individual to actively seek support: "I've walked away from them I suppose . . . they haven't fallen out of contact with me, I've fallen out of contact with them" or the perception that there was no valid reason to expect support: "I haven't really got an excuse to invite friends over." Turner et al. (2007) similarly found that some individuals isolated themselves during the transition from hospital to home, so the current findings are not surprising.

Types of Support Needed
The data confirmed the existence of a distinction between emotional, practical, and information based support as outlined by the majority of social support researchers and theorists (Cutrona & Russell, 1990; Due, Holstein, Lund, Modvig, & Avlund, 1999; McColl et al., 1995). Information based support included providing or obtaining education about brain injury, information about a range of topics including employment and educational options, services and financial assistance, social opportunities and daily activities, situation-specific advice and suggestions, and feedback regarding performance or behavior. As one person stated, "I really needed someone to tell me what to do because I didn't know."

Emotional support was defined as the provision of reassurance, being there when needed, encouragement, companionship and conversation, listening and understanding, empathy, having faith, hope and optimism, realistic expectations, showing an interest, friendship, provision of personal space, patience, affection and intimacy, acceptance and respect, and avoidance of patronizing and blame as well as allowing self-direction. Descriptions of emotional support also included, "To know that I was of use to somebody . . . would be the reassurance I needed" and

> I think just understanding because there's nothing they can do or anybody can do, just understanding goes a hell of a long way . . . please accept us as we are, things happen, I'm a little bit different, I don't want to be comforted, but I just want the understanding.

As found by Rotondi and colleagues (2007), people with ABI need family, friends, and coworkers to have a better understanding of what they were going through and a need to be accepted as they are. Affirmation was important: "What I've found comes from my social network and from my wife is affirmation on what I'm doing." People indicated that they would prefer to receive emotional support from friends rather than family or professionals: "Just people being there and helping me out when I need it and talking to me and listening . . . I never get that from my friends really." Paradoxically however, friends were commonly a source of negative impact: "I became an outcast in my own friends. I just lost all my friends basically. They didn't, they wouldn't come around, when they saw what I was and what I'd turned into, and they couldn't cope with it. . . ."

Practical supports included the provision of vocational, physical, and cognitive skills; assistance with activities of daily living; assistance with planning things and providing prompts and reminders, financial assistance, advocacy, and problem-solving; collaborative decision-making; counseling, recognition, and avoidance of negative triggers; back-up in unfamiliar situations; and participation and assistance in educational and recreational activities and social outings. As one person stated, "I don't expect people to pay for me. But a little bit of financial support from at times when I need it would be good. But I do get that . . . mum and dad." Another stated: "I keep coming in at least once a week to drop my washing back in, because mum is nice enough to do my washing for me." Practical support was preferred to be received from professionals and family rather than friends and informational support was preferred from professionals rather than family or friends: "I really think that some counseling and professional help would have been good . . . some training and education," and "very quickly you can lose your direction . . . some community support like that . . . family and friends, it's hard to take notice of them." The distinction between emotional support from friends and informational support from professionals was articulated by one person:

> Friends need to support me and push me a little but I will need some knowledgeable person to help me organize . . . I don't know where to start so that person could show me where I can get volunteer work and education and help me do the paperwork.

Strandberg (2009) highlighted that this type of professional support is essential following ABI. Families actually provided more practical support than either friends or professionals, a finding supported by Turner et al. (2007). Families often provided support that was perceived to be more appropriate coming from other sources:

> Mum would be the best person because I see her all time. With emotions, probably a partner would be good. Like mum could do that but would be more a spouse . . . she does that because I don't have a partner, she hasn't got much choice really.

Strandberg (2009) suggested that more often than not, a decrease in friends and relationships resulted in complimentary increases in family support.

Friends provided more emotional support than practical support, although there were instances where practical support was provided: "I had some friends that realized what the problem was, and they'd come and pick me up and take me to parties and things." However, information based support was not provided at all by friends. Professionals were most likely to provide practical assistance and information. Younger people ideally required and tended to receive more emotional support from friends than older people whereas older people required more practical support from family, indicating that the acceptability of family support was clearly related to age.

> I get the support I need in those situations from the family now . . .
> I think maybe it is a maturity thing as well, maybe as we get older we become more accepting of other people and we accept them with their limitations . . .

However, many people referred to the need for age-appropriate support: "You do boring shit, like mum and dad shit, you know, I'm just way not interested in." In general, the primary type of support required by females was emotional support whereas for males, this was practical support. Similarly, partnered people required more practical support whereas unpartnered people required more emotional support. Not surprisingly, partnered people preferred to receive more support from family members and also reported receiving more support from family members. Unpartnered people reported receiving significantly more support from professionals. In contrast to the required types of support, practical support was the most common type of support actually received and information based support was received least frequently. Family support was most frequently received in response to tangible issues, friend support was most frequently received in relationship issues, and professional support was most frequently received to assist with achievement. Some people disliked how they received different support for different situations at different times.

Matching Support to Needs

Typically, there was a poor match between ideal and actual levels of support for people with ABI. Indeed, when people described the degree to which their support needs had been met, support was generally insufficient in either quantity or quality. Across all vignettes and people (i.e., 16 vignettes by 15 people—240 responses), in only eight responses did people believe their needs had been met by their current network. Only four people accounted for these eight responses. Three of the four people were older males, two of whom were married. Two of these people had experienced only a small number of the vignettes relative to the rest of the sample. For instance, one older married male had experienced only four of the 16 situations. Another older married male had experienced only three vignettes and for all three, there was a match between ideal and actual support. He stated, "my family and friends provide me with all the support that I need."

There were four ways in which support was considered inadequate. First, some people did not receive the amount of support that they needed: "Well when I see them [friends] like [they] . . . make me feel more normal but, yeah, don't see them that often so it isn't normal . . . not like before." Some stated that friends were not prepared to make effort: "Out of 100 friends, four of them made an effort" and others stated that they were not confident enough to ask for support: "Rather than me being assertive, they have to ask me now, whereas once upon a time, I'd have asserted what I felt." Lamontagne and colleagues (2009) suggested that, for young ABI survivors, human assistance requires continual daily efforts and adjustments from both parties.

Second, people indicated that they had received support, but not the type they were seeking. For example, one person stated, "Sometimes you just need some encouragement . . . not somebody to do it for you. I am not completely useless." Similarly another person stated, "Family should be the ones who are there to help you out the most . . . they might be trying to help me in their own way, but it's not the way I want them to help." Often, people felt they had to educate others to ensure they provided appropriate support: "It's always a little bit difficult acquainting people with your problem, educating people about your needs." Others felt they had to ask for support: "You can't assume that everybody will know what to do and then other people don't care . . . but you have to ask."

Third, the source of support was often considered inappropriate to meet the needs of the individual. For instance, one person stated that

> Like before I wouldn't always go out with my family. I would spend most of my weekends with my friends and maybe only see my family for an hour or so . . . but now it is like everywhere with my family . . . and that is good but it isn't the same.

Another example was provided by one person who reported, "And it is real good to be with those people [other people with ABI] . . . because they understand where you have been . . . But it is not like they can really be good friends."

Fourth, some people described support that was negative and actually created conflict. Negative support was described in the following ways: "Your friends, they don't want to know you . . . they only see you when they want something. Like I bet when I get my money they will all be my mates again" or, "and when I ask the kids to do something they sort of laugh, as if to say oh mum can't read that or mum can't do this." Labeling was common: "[Family] Put labels on me, you know I'm a bitch, I act weird, you know I'm temperamental, I'm impatient, I treat my kids dah, dah, dah . . ." as was criticism, "criticized to my face. My family behind my back discussing my terrible behavior, or how dare I act like that." "They humiliate you, abuse you, and then when you get upset, they blame you." Reichard, Langlois, Sample, Wald, and Pickelsimer (2007) studied violence, abuse, and neglect in nine people with ABI and found that negative support was not usually a discrete event but was cumulative in daily life, created by vulnerability and cognitive impairments and perpetrated by many different people across an individual's network.

Across all responses to all vignettes, negative support was mentioned in 105 of the 240 responses. Only one person (an older married male) did not report any negative support. In many cases, the support required by the person involved cessation of support that was causing distress: "Don't be overprotective and treat me like a baby" or "My 'olds' should let me make my own mistakes." The family was often the most common source of negative support: "I still do have family problems, because my mum is not letting me go out." Even among older people with good support: "They are extremely supportive of me and probably sometimes I might think that they are a bit over supportive, 'oh you shouldn't be doing that dad.'" Gauvin-Lepage and Lefebvre (2010) found that overprotectiveness commonly occurred among parents and this may strengthen or weaken support systems in the family.

As one person stated, "[The support required] depends on the situation . . . It would have to be somebody in that situation, who knows the situation and they can say like do this and do that and give me alternatives on different ways to do things." Emotional support was the primary type of support required in the majority of vignettes except for those related to tangible tasks such as shopping. In these instances, practical support and support from professionals was most frequently required: "Support from family and friends, they just were not acquainted with this . . . a rather specialist subject . . . you do need a bit of specialist care in rehabilitation." Family support was considered important for achievement and role functioning: "It's hard to find time because of the kids. I tried a sport but it just didn't work out. I had no-one to look after them for me while I played"; whereas friend support was necessary for relationship issues. Many situations required combined types of support from multiple sources. For instance, difficulties with memory required both practical and emotional support from family and friends as well as informational support from professionals. Practical support in terms of prompting needed to be coupled with emotional support in terms of understanding: "Need them to act as a reminder. Like if you said that you would be meeting them at such and such a time and you might forget, they will need to give you a call and remind you"; "Probably not getting snappy because I told you this yesterday . . . understand that my short term memory is . . . they get upset because I've forgotten something." Ironically, some described how their lack of success in daily situations was likely to increase their lack of support, creating a downward spiral of support: "Most of it comes down to like, you can't get jobs, you haven't got friends, you can't get relationships, so the hole just, it's like you're digging yourself a hole deeper and deeper."

Communication about Support

Some people spoke of the difficulties they experienced receiving support due to lack of inhibition or other changes in their personality and behavior: "I started an unnecessary conversation and thought he had gone very quiet all of a sudden. I just got carried away, he'd just hung up while I was babbling away, he just quietly put the phone down." "I have a volatile personality now. I don't get violent, but I get outspoken . . . like my own way of saying something, rather than waiting until someone else has had their say first." Others spoke about difficulty participating in supportive interactions when people could not understand them: "I couldn't speak properly . . . when I was talking I knew that no way no one would understand what I was saying . . . I think I knew what I was thinking, but I knew I wasn't saying it correctly." Similarly, cognitive disabilities inhibited supportive interactions: "I've been involved with a few relationships and not one of them understands the difficulty just having a conversation, trying to keep your mind on what you're talking about." Donovan-Kicken and

Bute (2008) noted that impaired communication often created uncertainty about diagnosis, level of understanding, and the expression of emotion. Informational support is essential in these situations. However, Roscigno and Van Liew (2008) highlighted that professional discourses often assume that faulty social interactions originate from the person with TBI. In this regard, it is important to note that cognitive impairments alone cannot completely explain social isolation following ABI, especially over time. Considerable effort is required on the part of support providers to ensure that they are providing appropriate support at appropriate times and in appropriate ways. However, considerable effort was also required on the part of people with ABI to ensure that their needs were communicated clearly and that they actively mobilized their support network when required.

Conclusion

The current findings demonstrate that people with ABI have specific needs for emotional, practical, and information based support depending on their particular experiences. Seeking social support is a contextual process that must match the demands of the environment or situation. A clearer understanding of the match between ideal and actual support may be the key to identifying effective interventions that will assist people with ABI to return to a life where they feel as though they are valued and important members of the community. This chapter has highlighted the importance of support and the benefits that can be derived from carefully crafted responses to different situations. However, it is also important to recognize the pressure experienced by family members and friends as they learn to manage the impact of ABI on their own lives. Under such circumstances, the ability to provide unconditional support is likely to be severely compromised, resulting in negative feelings on the part of both the person with ABI and his or her family and friends. There is clearly a critical role for professionals to do more than simply assume a central role in the support network of people with ABI. Instead, the elevated role of professionals in the support network offers them a unique opportunity to acknowledge the needs of both parties and the importance of natural supports. In doing so, they can actively facilitate the successful match between support needs and the delivery of supportive actions over time.

References

Coyne, J. C., Ellard, J. H., & Smith, D. A. (1990). Social support, independence and the dilemmas of helping. In I. G. Sarason, B. R. Sarason, & G. R. Pierce (Eds.), *Social support: an interactional view* (pp. 129–149). New York: Wiley.

Cutrona, C. E., & Russell, D. (1990). Type of social support and specific stress: Toward a theory of optimal matching. In I. G. Sarason, B. R. Sarason, & G. R. Pierce (Eds.), *Social support: an interactional view* (pp. 319–366). New York: Wiley.

Cutrona, C. E., & Suhr, J. A. (1992). Controllability of stressful events and satisfaction with spouse support behaviors. *Communication Research, 19*(2), 154–174.

Degeneffe, C. E., & Lee, G. K. (2010). Quality of life after traumatic brain injury: Perspectives of adult siblings. *Journal of Rehabilitation, 76*(4), 27–36.

Doig, E., Fleming, J., Cornwell, P., & Kuipers, P. (2011). Comparing the experience of outpatient therapy in home and day hospital settings after traumatic brain injury: Patient, significant other and therapist perspectives. *Disability and Rehabilitation, 33*(13–14), 1203–14.

Donovan-Kicken, E., & Bute J. J. (2008). Uncertainty of social network members in the case of communication-debilitating illness or injury. *Qualitative Health Research, 18*(1), 5–18.

Due, P., Holstein, B., Lund, R., Modvig, J., & Avlund, K. (1999). Social relations: Network, support and relational strain. *Social Science & Medicine, 48*(5), 661–673.

Elsass, L., & Kinsella, G. (1987). Social interaction following severe closed head injury. *Psychological Medicine, 17*(1), 67–78.

Finset, A., Dyrnes, S., Krogstad, J. M., & Berstad, J. (1995). Self-reported social networks and interpersonal support 2 years after severe traumatic brain injury. *Brain Injury, 9*(2), 141–150.

Gauvin-Lepage, J., & Lefebvre, H. (2010). Social inclusion of persons with moderate head injuries: the points of view of adolescents with brain injuries, their parents and professionals. *Brain Injury, 24*(9), 1087–1097.

Gill, C. J., Sander, A.M., Robins, N., Mazzei, D. K., & Struchen, M. A. (2011). Exploring experiences of intimacy from the viewpoint of individuals with traumatic brain injury and their partners. *Journal of Head Trauma Rehabilitation, 26*(1), 56–68.

Glass, T. A., & Maddox, G. L. (1992). The quality and quantity of social support: Stroke recovery as psychosocial transition. *Social Science & Medicine, 34*(11), 1249–1261.

Jacobson, D. E. (1986). Types and timing of social support. *Journal of Health and Social Behavior, 27*(3), 250–264.

Kozloff, R. (1987). Networks of social support and the outcome from severe head injury. *Journal of Head Trauma Rehabilitation, 2*(3), 14–23.

Kreutzer, J. S., Marwitz, J. H., & Kepler, K. (1992). Traumatic brain injury: Family response and outcome. *Archives of Physical Medicine and Rehabilitation, 73*(8), 771–778.

Lamontagne, M-E., Ouellet, M-C., & Simard, J-F. (2009). A descriptive portrait of human assistance required by individuals with brain injury. *Brain Injury, 23*(7–8), 693–701.

Lefebvre, H., Cloutier, G., & Levert, M. J. (2008). Perspectives of survivors of traumatic brain injury and their caregivers on long-term social integration. *Brain Injury, 22*(7–8), 535–543.

McColl, M. A., Lei, H., & Skinner, H. (1995). Structural relationships between social support and coping. *Social Science & Medicine, 41*(3), 395–407.

Minnes, P., Woodford, L., Carlson, P., Johnston, J., & McColl, M. A. (2010). The needs of aging parents caring for an adult with acquired brain injury. *Canadian Journal on Aging / Revue Canadienne Du Vieillissement, 29*(2), 185–192.

Muenchberger, H., Sunderland, N., Kendall, E., & Quinn, H. (2011). A long way to tipperary? Young people with complex health conditions living in residential aged care: a metaphorical map for understanding the call for change. *Disability and Rehabilitation, 33*(13–14), 1190–1202.

Paterson, J., & Stewart, J. (2002). Adults with acquired brain injury: Perceptions of their social world. *Rehabilitation Nursing, 27*(1), 13–18.

Pruchno, R. A., Patrick, J. H., & Burant, C. J. (1996). Aging women and their children with chronic disabilities–Perceptions of sibling involvement and effects on well-being. *Family Relations, 45*(3), 318–326.

Reichard, A. A., Langlois, J. A., Sample, P. L., Wald, M. M., & Pickelsimer, E. E. (2007). Violence, abuse, and neglect among people with traumatic brain injuries. *Journal of Head Trauma Rehabilitation, 22*(6), 390–402.

Robison, J., Wiles, R., Ellis-Hill, C., McPherson, K., Hyndman, D., & Ashburn, A. (2009). Resuming previously valued activities post-stroke: Who or what helps? *Disability and Rehabilitation, 31*(19), 1555–1566.

Roscigno, C. I., & Van Liew, K. (2008). Pushed to the margins and pushing back: a case study of one adult's reflections on social interactions after a traumatic brain injury sustained as an adolescent. *Journal of Neuroscience Nursing, 40*(4), 212–221.

Rotondi, A. J., Sinkule, J., Balzer, K., Harris, J., & Moldovan, R. (2007). A qualitative needs assessment of persons who have experienced traumatic brain injury and their primary family caregivers. *Journal of Head Trauma Rehabilitation, 22*(1), 14–25.

Seeman, T. E., & Berkman, L. F. (1988). Structural characteristics of social networks and their relationship with social support in the elderly: Who provides support. *Social Science & Medicine, 26*(7), 737–749.

Strandberg, T. (2009). Adults with acquired traumatic brain injury: Experiences of a changeover process and consequences in everyday life. *Social Work in Health Care, 48*(3), 276–297.

Struchen, M. A., Davis, L. C., Bogaards, J. A., Hudler-Hull, T., Clark, A. N., Mazzei, D. M., . . . Caroselli, J. S. (2011). Making connections after brain injury: Development and evaluation of a social peer-mentoring program for persons with traumatic brain injury. *Journal of Head Trauma Rehabilitation, 26*(1), 4–19.

Swift, T. L., & Wilson, S. L. (2001). Misconceptions about brain injury among the general public and non-expert health professionals: an exploratory study. *Brain Injury, 15*(2), 149–165.

Tomberg, T., Toomela, A., Ennok, M., & Tikk, A. (2007). Changes in coping strategies, social support, optimism and health-related quality of life following traumatic brain injury: a longitudinal study. *Brain Injury, 21*(5), 479–488.

Turner, B., Fleming, J., Cornwell, P., Worrall, L., Ownsworth, T., Haines, T., Kendall, M., & Chenoweth, L. (2007). A qualitative study of the transition from hospital to home for individuals with acquired brain injury and their family caregivers. *Brain Injury, 21*(11), 1119–1130.

Willer, B., & Corrigan, J. D. (1994). Whatever it takes: a model for community-based services. *Brain Injury, 8*(7), 647–659.

Zencius, A. H., & Wesolowski, M. D. (1999). Is the social network analysis necessary in the rehabilitation of individuals with head injury? *Brain Injury, 13*(9), 723–727.

CHAPTER 6

Too Small for Your Boots! Understanding the Experience of Children When Family Members Acquire a Neurological Condition

Samantha Bursnall and Kenneth I. Pakenham

Young people who provide care for a family member who has a disability are often referred to as young carers or young care givers in the United States. Over the last decade, an increasing amount of research has examined the responsibilities these young people are likely to assume as a result of their role as a carer (Aldridge & Becker, 1993; Newman, 2002; Olsen, 1996). Although this literature has been invaluable in lifting the profile of young carers and raising awareness about their needs, little is still known about *how* they experience their situation and its impact on their young lives. This chapter proposes a framework that offers some depth, context, and meaning within which our knowledge about these young people can be progressed.

Many young carers remain unrecognized and *hidden* in the community without appropriate support (Becker, 2007; Dearden & Becker, 2004). Recent research has indicated that the number of youngsters who assume a caring role is likely to increase in future due to advances in health technology, health care system changes, the aging population, changes in family structures (e.g., increases in sole parent households), policy shifts (e.g., deinstitutionalization), and an increase in the number of people living with disabilities (Aldridge & Becker, 1993; Olsen, 1996). Although little is known about this population, one widely agreed upon characteristic of young carers is that they are young people who assume exaggerated levels of responsibility that may have a negative impact on their own development (Aldridge & Becker, 1999). For example, it has been suggested that they may be at increased risk of poor physical and mental health, impaired psychosocial development, low participation rates in education, restricted opportunities to access vocational training, financial insecurity, and lack of independence (Aldridge & Becker, 1999; Cree, 2003; Dearden & Becker, 2004; Olsen, 1996). In addition, it has been suggested that caring is responsible for limitations on their ability to participate in social activities, employment, relationships, and recreation (Dearden & Becker, 2004).

Ironically, these young people may already be vulnerable given the factors that contribute to their likelihood of becoming young carers are similar to those that contribute to other forms of social disadvantage (e.g., the perception that they have little or no choice) (Aldridge, 2006; Banks et al., 2002; Bolas, Van Wersch, & Flynn, 2007; Pakenham, Bursnall, Chiu, Cannon, & Okochi, 2006); poverty, single-parent households, a lack of appropriate services, and deinstitutionalization (Aldridge, 2006; Becker, 2007; Shifren & Kachorek, 2003). In a full review of current research focused on young carers, Pakenham (2009) outlines many more impacts and negative consequences of their role.

Although several large-scale surveys and systematic reviews have been conducted (Pakenham et al., 2006; Pakenham & Bursnall, 2006; Pakenham, Chiu, Bursnall, & Cannon, 2007), they have been largely descriptive and have relied on youth selected from clinical or welfare populations who are already receiving support, thus may not be representative of young carers in general (Cree, 2003; Dearden & Becker, 2004; Newman, 2002). With the exception of one study conducted by Metzing-Blau and Schnepp (2008) that explored the young carer experience from a systemic family-oriented perspective, a notable shortfall of past research is that it has failed to provide a framework from which to understand *how* and *why* having a parent with a disability impacts on youngsters. The lack of conceptual models that tie together the many issues identified by researchers limits the ability of health professionals to provide appropriate interventions to support these children. Such shortcomings are likely to stem from the reductionist approach that is inherent in many of the studies to date. These studies are based on the selection of clinical samples using predetermined definitions of what constitutes a young carer. The broad clinical outcome measures that are often used in young carer research are likely to lack sensitivity to issues relevant to this population (Pakenham et al., 2006).

To address some of these shortcomings, this chapter examines pertinent issues from the perspective of young carers with the intention of building a conceptual model that contextualizes their many disparate experiences. Given that children do not always identify themselves as *carers*, as well as the lack of available evidence regarding the characteristics and roles of these youngsters, the recruitment process in this study did not require them to self identify as young carers. Instead, this chapter focuses only on the experiences of people (children and adults) who, when between the ages of 9 and 13 years, had a parent with an acquired neurological condition (see Table 6.1). This age range was chosen to reflect the likelihood that the young people were old enough to be engaged in daily chores but not old enough to live independently. It was also important to obtain retrospective views from adult participants who were no longer actively involved in caregiving because they can reflect on their past experiences (Miles & Huberman, 1984). Although the recipients of care are sometimes siblings, and to a lesser extent, a grandparent or other adult relative outside the immediate family (Newman, 2002), the greatest impact of caring is likely to be found when the recipient of care is a parent (Dearden & Becker, 1998, 2004; Worsham, Compass, & Sydney, 1997). Thus, the focus of this chapter is on children caring for their parents.

Eight young Australian people were interviewed (2 males, 6 females) who were aged 9 to 37 years. Three of the participants were adults aged between 25 and 37 who had cared for their parent as a child, and five were children at the time of the interview (aged 9 to 13 years). All participants had a parent who had an acquired neurological disability. The young people lived with both parents, although two of the adults no longer lived at home. None were receiving formal support services at the time of their interview. A second group of six young carers (4 males, 2 females) living in the United Kingdom were also interviewed. This group of young carers differed from the original sample in that they lived in a different country (the West Midlands in the UK) and cared for different family members who had different types of disabilities. Unlike the initial group in Australia, these UK young carers did identify themselves as young carers and belonged to a Young Carer Support Group. Aged between 13 and 19 years, two participants cared for their mothers, three for a sibling, and one had cared for both parents and two siblings before

Table 6.1 Summary of participant and parental characteristics

Parental Condition	Participants		Father	Mother
	N	Age range	N	N
Acquired brain injury (ABI)	3	9–13	1	2
Epilepsy	2	12–13	0	2
Huntington's disease (HD)	1	25	0	1
Mental Illness	2	35–39	0	2
Total	8	9–39	1	7

they died. The neurological illnesses and disabilities of care-recipients included epilepsy, cerebella ataxia, attention-deficit and hyperactivity disorder, and an additional diagnosis of cancer. These young people had been caring for their family member for at least 3 years. Thus, this chapter reflects the views of young caregivers across two countries, a range of disabilities, numerous family circumstances, and different support networks.

The Adult Child—A Central Theme

A conceptual model was generated from the interviews (see Figure 6.1). The model indicates that caregiving presented a number of emotional issues for children, regardless of whether or not they undertook direct

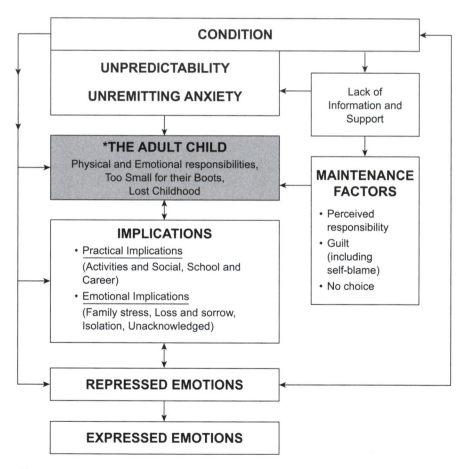

Figure 6.1 The adult child: too small for your boots. A model representing the core experiences of children who care for a parent with an illness/disability. *Shaded to depict core category.

physical caring responsibilities. Elements of their parents' condition led children to perceive disability as being *unpredictable* and uncertain, which in turn led them to feel *unremitting anxiety* and concern. The lack of information and appropriate support appeared to exacerbate this process.

A central theme that emerged from this data was that of the *adult child*, which described the process in which the young people engaged to manage and minimize the impact (i.e., unpredictability and unremitting anxiety) of their parents' condition. Specifically, participants undertook a number of emotional and physical caring tasks traditionally reserved for adults. Several factors appeared to influence and maintain this role including: (1) the perception that they had control over and responsibility for their parents' recovery, (2) guilt, and (3) no choice but to help. Again, a lack of information, and appropriate support appeared to fuel these feelings. Although the young people became adult children, they indicated that they were not always comfortable with this role, and metaphorically described the feeling of being *too small for their boots* and regretful of their *lost childhood*. As depicted in the model, this role as an adult child was central to, accounted for, and linked with all other categories.

Not surprisingly, the young people experienced a number of practical and emotional implications because of their parents' condition and their adult roles and responsibilities. The practical implications included a disruption to their activities and social lives, school, and careers. The emotional implications included a mix of emotions, such as family stress, isolation, and feeling a lack of acknowledgment. They reported that they tended to repress their feelings, which in turn, appeared to maintain the status quo. Young people who expressed emotions, however, had the opportunity to gain perspective on, relief from, and support in their role as an adult child. Each of these themes that emerged from the data is described below.

The Experience of Caregiving

Type of Illness or Condition. Although the neurological conditions young people dealt with differed in terms of onset, diagnosis, prognosis, and symptomatology, there were similarities in the nature of the conditions and the impact these had on the young people. Specifically, all the young people reported that the illness trajectory of their parent's condition had elements of unpredictability and uncertainty, even if they had learned how to predict the condition to some extent. Unpredictability of the condition related to many factors, including traumatic onset of the illness/disability (e.g., traumatic brain injury/stroke), unpredictable periodic onset of symptoms, and/or on-going changes to the parent's condition (e.g., deterioration). One young person described the nature of her mother's schizophrenia as, ". . . being tearful one minute and having any emotion the next, it was like a roller-coaster ride . . ."

The ongoing unpredictability and vulnerability of their parents' health naturally caused the young people unremitting anxiety and concern. Even when an illness/disability was relatively stable or in remission, the possibility of its return meant that the young people's anxiety and worry never fully abated. This meant that they were alert and hypersensitive to the possibility of recurrences of the condition.

> Like most days in the morning, I think "Is she going to have a fit? What's going to happen?'. . . I think about it like every day, sort of. All I can remember is like blood all over her face [when she hit her face falling from a fit], bleeding mouth, her screaming when the ambulance came. (Young carer)

When asked what would be different if her mum did not have epilepsy, one young person replied:

> We wouldn't be sad, we wouldn't be worried; we would feel safe all the time because it wouldn't matter. She would walk to school without us thinking, is she going to have [an episode]? When is it going to happen?

Lack of Information and Inclusion. The unpredictability, confusion, and uncertainty experienced by the young people often related to a general lack of information and support regarding their parent's condition in terms of the diagnosis, prognosis, and treatment: "No one has really come and explained it to me . . ." It was common for the young people to be excluded from the planning of their parent's treatment. Most of the young people were not provided with information about what to expect or how to manage their parents' condition. Privacy laws precluded one young person from accessing information about her mother's illness.

There also seemed to be a lack of understanding from the community and service providers about the needs and issues faced by the young people: "you care about this person so much . . . but you are young enough that people won't listen to you or understand what you need." As shown in Figure 7.1 and discussed below, a lack of information contributed to the maintenance of factors such as unpredictability, unremitting anxiety, adult child role, perceived responsibility, guilt, no choice, and repressed emotions.

The Adult Child. As mentioned earlier, most of the young people expressed that the unpredictable nature of their parent's condition and their consequent anxiety led them to shoulder physical and emotional responsibilities to care for their parent; such responsibilities were beyond those usually expected of children. One young person explained, "You end up being the adult. The adult child." The data indicated that participants undertook a series of physical care responsibilities, such as personal care duties, including showering, dressing, and medicating their parent, particularly when their parent had physical limitations. Physical responsibilities also extended to everyday household chores, such as laundry, cooking, caring for siblings, budgeting, and paying bills. Emotional care responsibilities included comforting the parent and monitoring their mental state that in two instances occurred just after being sent home from a suicide attempt. One UK teenager said, "yes I agree, because it is like being an adult in a child's body. You're not living a child's life and doing what other children do."

Although the young people indicated that they adopted the adult role because they perceived themselves to be responsible for their parents' well-being, they felt guilt, and/or believed there to be no other options. They did not necessarily feel comfortable in this role. Many felt they were "too small for their boots." "It was more of a dumped in the big end. . . . You can't step into shoes, you know, ten sizes bigger than yours without feeling really uncomfortable and needing to be guided." Similarly, when asked how they felt about being responsible much of the time, one 12-year-old said, "You don't want to do that—be older than your years."

Indeed, many younger adults reflected that they had a lost childhood, "I feel like I have missed out on so much and put so much on hold. . . . I would really like to just start living my life." When the adults were no longer in the caring role, it appeared that they had permission to observe and acknowledge the many childhood experiences they missed out on that the younger children did not yet verbalize.

> I didn't feel much about that then, [but] as I get older and the more I think . . . back on those issues I grieve for my lost childhood now. At the time I really wasn't aware that was happening but with hindsight I can see that is what happened. (Young adult carer)

This adult role appeared to be maintained by perceived responsibility, guilt, and limited choice about the caring role, which were exacerbated by a lack of information and support.

Maintenance Factors

Perceived Responsibility. Implicit in the young people's language was a strong sense of responsibility for and perceived control over their parent's recovery, which appears to have influenced and maintained their responsible behavior. They expressed a responsibility to be available to their parent at all times: "I feel like I have to be close to her all the time in case something happens," and the associated relentlessness, as described by one 13-year-old: "I feel I deserve a break, but I worry if she is going to be okay. So if I have a break I end up calling every five minutes to check. The responsibility doesn't end."

Guilt. Guilt appeared to be the first response that the young people experienced if they did not fulfill the carer role: ". . . I used to just go out . . . But I would always be feeling guilty for doing so." Guilt was so strong that many participants sacrificed their own needs and desires to care for their parent. Guilt also appeared in the form of self-blame, with many people believing that they had somehow caused their parent's disability: "Sometimes I feel so angry that I hit myself . . . I feel like it is my fault . . . Like [the germ] got on me and then went on mummy . . ." Self-blame often went hand-in-hand with a lack of information about the causes and conditions of the parents' condition.

No Choice, All Responsibility. The responsibilities undertaken by the young people were maintained because they perceived there to be no other option for them: ". . . Nobody said that I had to do it, it was kind of something I took on. . . . There is nobody else to do it so you have to," and "If I don't do it, who's going to?" Not surprisingly, lack of information, support (for parents and their children) and perceived inadequate service provision maintained the young people's perception that they had control, responsibility, and little choice about adopting the carer role, "the hospital said to me 'sorry you are just going to have to take her home. . .' There was no explanation from doctors or nurses . . . they basically washed their hands of her." Some young carers believed that they provided the best level of care to their parents and that acquiring help was actually more stressful if not of a good standard, thus reinforcing the adult role.

Practical Implications

Social Impact. Most young people mentioned that their social lives were affected as a result of their parent's condition or the caring role. Many missed extracurricular activities because they were required to help their parent or because their activities were not a family priority. Some avoided engaging with friends due to concerns about being embarrassed by their parent's behavior, "I always tried to keep my friends away from the house. . ."

School and Career. Not surprisingly, their responsibilities also affected some young people's schooling and consequently their career opportunities, due to either the caring role or the inability to concentrate due to worry, for instance, one young carer explained, "I can't get everything . . . done so I have to ask the teachers for extensions." And another reported,

> I used to spend probably one day a week off school to do the house-work. I never really went through high school. Primary school, I think I was there, but concentrating when you've got that—you

can't. . . . School is not important when you know you've got to go home and watch the place and survive with less food . . . school's not a priority. (Young carer)

Family Impact. Although some young people described that as a result of their parent's illness/disability they became closer to family members, others experienced stress and family conflict in the home as a result of the illness/disability and the associated caring role. Most young people described a mixture of experiences that ranged from closeness to conflict, "Since [the illness], I have fallen apart from him [father] a bit. . . . Me and mum have had a couple of fights and we never really had fights [before father's illness]." In some situations, the caring role put further strain on relationships when it was shared, which lead to conflict and stress in the home: "We have completely different caring styles. . . . I still do [care for mum] but not as much because Dad and I start fighting about it a bit . . . "

Isolation. One of the most common feelings described by all of the young people was a sense of isolation. They described feeling isolated from other people because they viewed their experience as exclusive and incomprehensible to anyone who had not been in similar circumstances "because it hasn't happened to them before." Desperation associated with not feeling understood was highlighted by one young person who said, "you wouldn't wish it on anyone, but you wish your friends could be in this situation just so they understand. Only someone who's been through it can understand."

Caring Is Work. Many young people felt unacknowledged and un-recognized in the caring experience: "People don't respect that caring is work." Some young people who cared for a parent were not recognized as a carer if a primary carer, such as a well parent, also lived in the home. There were other feelings of loss described by young carers. Loss and sorrow reflected a culmination of factors including the nature of their parents' condition, their care-giving role, or changes in their parent following their illness.

> I remember being . . . sad. Just sad that, I guess in my heart I knew there was something wrong, I knew particular things were . . . wrong and I was sad that my brothers and sisters weren't doing what kids should be doing . . .

Emotional Expression. Most of the young people, despite feeling such an array of emotions, did not express their feelings. This was largely due to their perceived isolation and the lack of understanding they felt from peers, family, and community, as well as a lack of knowledge of appropriate support services. Many did not perceive themselves to be eligible for support or did not know where to access it, "at the peak of mum's illness . . . I didn't know what to do, where to turn, and so I just handled it all inwardly." The young people interviewed were also reluctant to talk to close friends and family for fear of burdening them, "[I don't talk to mum] because . . . I think I would be bothering her." Not expressing their feelings and concerns effectively made them invisible to assistance and ultimately maintained the emotional and practical impact of their situation.

However, some young people said that they eventually expressed their feelings to some friends even if their friends did not know how to help. In terms of support, the young people were clear that they wanted their friends "to listen to you, not feel sorry for you." Talking to friends helped to "get it off my chest [so] I can do everything again" as explained by a young carer. Generally, they advocated that expressing their fears, frustration, and concerns was cathartic, "we just talked about it and she made me feel a little bit better." Further, talking appeared to increase their chances of accessing support. Once support was accessed, it was perceived to be helpful in breaking free of the implications and the cycle perpetuating their repressed thoughts and feelings. "Once you tap in, everyone's very well at making sure you are linked into everything that is available . . ."

Conclusion

Overall, young carers in active caring roles across two continents assumed the role of the *adult child*, in which they undertook an unusually high level of physical and emotional responsibilities. Earley and Cushway (2002) similarly referred to this role as the parental child. They argued that such role reversal was inappropriate and had potential to disrupt the balance of the family system and negatively impact on children's development. Although this negative impact may be the case, removing the child from the caring role may actually be detrimental to the youngsters involved as the role often enables them to abate their worries, fears, guilt, and concerns. In this regard, our study has supported Aldridge and Becker's (1996) suggestion that respect should be granted to young people who wish to be involved in the care of their parent but that they should be adequately supported in that role.

A great deal of research examining the impact of caregiving on the psychological adjustment of young people has suggested that these youngsters require ongoing emotional support, particularly through the period of caregiving. For instance, Banks et al. (2001) found that youngsters caring for a relative reported higher depression and lower self-esteem than non-carers. Another study that investigated the long-term effects of early caregiving found that up to 75 percent of young carers developed psychological problems as adults, especially if their care recipients had challenging behaviors, mental illnesses, or alcohol/drug-related problems (Frank,

Tatum, & Tucker, 1999). More recently, Pakenham et al. (2006) found that compared to non-carers, young carers reported significantly higher levels of adverse caregiving impacts, less reliance on problem-solving coping, higher somatization, and lower life satisfaction.

The young people interviewed were profoundly affected by the unpredictable nature of their parent's condition and the unremitting anxiety that resulted. Several researchers have suggested that the long-term prognosis of a disability is likely to be as important in anticipating the future challenges of young carers, as the caring role itself (Olsen, 1996; Rolland, 1999). Metzing-Blau and Schnepp (2008) highlighted how the unpredictable nature of some disabilities, such as those associated with neurological (cognitive and emotional) conditions, keeps these children on high alert, "ready to act at any time."

Best research and practice ought to consider the impact of a variety of contextual factors on youngsters whose parent is disabled, including the psychological impact of the nature and prognosis of the condition, as well as the needs of young carers that arise from the caring tasks themselves. Indeed, Metzing-Blau and Schnepp (2008) suggested that quality supportive interventions involve the entire family, especially since children need not be shielded against parental disability and, in fact, may wish to help more effectively where they can. Their capacity to help effectively (and cope better themselves) is likely to be associated with the extent to which they understand and can predict the consequences of the parental condition.

Although not generalizable across all services dealing with young carers, the lack of support and information affecting these young carers impacted heavily on all areas of their caring role. It increased their anxiety and contributed to their perception that they had no choice but to take on the adult role. This perceived absence of choice led to practical and emotional fatigue, isolation, feeling misunderstood, a lack of knowledge about available supports, and reluctance to further burden their family. Sadly, these factors hid the children from any potential support system. Bolas et al. (2007) suggested that what isolates carers from being understood, recognized, and supported is their tendency to "maintain [their] invisibility by being secretive about their roles as carers, [which is] motivated by perceived stigma" and negative judgment (p. 839). According to Metzing-Blau and Schnepp (2008), silence and secrecy is a strategy used by these children to keep their family together and avoid being viewed as different, feeling misunderstood, or risk being separated. The danger of this situation, however, is that it maintains a cycle of isolation as the family closes ranks to protect its system (Metzing-Blau & Schnepp, 2008). Indeed, isolation and stigma are associated with poorer outcomes for young carers (Pakenham et al., 2006; Pakenham & Cox, 2012).

There is no doubt that this group of young people was similar to many other groups of young people: a mix of positive and negative states at any time, using vastly different coping strategies at different times in their lives and adjusting in different ways. If asked to rate them on a set of qualities, there would be a predictable mix of outcomes, some positive and some negative. This chapter focused on the experience of caring as perceived by the young carers themselves both at the time of the experience and with the benefit of hindsight. When asked to reflect on this experience and its impact on their lives, there was a tendency to focus on the challenges that caregiving presented. However, young carers also reported the use of critical strategies that enabled them to manage their situation. They had adopted new perspectives that had served them well despite the loss that pervaded their lives.

This chapter has highlighted the qualitative impact of caregiving on young people and raises important questions for service providers in future. For instance, how do service providers best respond to the multitude of potential factors that can have an impact on youngsters who have a parent with a disability? What information and support is required at particular points in the caring journey? How do young people stay "young" and enjoy childhood despite the caregiving role? How can services better respond to parents with disabilities to mitigate the impact of caregiving on their child? It is likely that providing appropriate and timely information will address many young carer concerns related to the prognosis and nature of their parent's condition. Importantly, however, Metzing-Blau and Schnepp (2008) highlighted that the way parents themselves coped impacted greatly on the experience of their children. For this reason, it is crucial that parents be helped to provide relief for young carers. Several studies have suggested the caring role may result in many benefits for young carers (Aldridge & Becker, 1993; Segal & Simkins, 1993), and the findings from this exploratory analysis indicate there are many other opportunities for intervention that can easily facilitate more positive experiences for young people, including their own health, identity, and wellbeing. Identifying the breadth and depth of issues is the first step in developing a more holistic response to the family disability experience. As individuals become increasingly informed about their own health condition and as new treatment and support options are realized in the future, it is anticipated that more appropriate resources will be identified and made available to this critical sub-population of unpaid carers.

Acknowledgments

This study was funded by a grant from the Ian Potter Foundation. We thank the generosity of participants in Australia and the Spurgeon's Young Carers Group in Wolverhampton, UK, for their time and involvement. Special thanks also to those in the community organizations who assisted with recruitment and Dr. Beven Yee for his comments. Great thanks also to Dr. Patricia Murphy for her useful input regarding the coding.

References

Aldridge, J. (2006). The experiences of children living with and caring for parents with mental illness. *Child Abuse Review, 15*(2), 79–88.

Aldridge, J., & Becker, S. (1993). *Children who care: Inside the world of young carers.* Loughborough: Young Carers Research Group.

Aldridge, J., & Becker, S. (1996). Disability rights and the denial of young carers: the dangers of zero-sum arguments. *Critical Social Policy, 16*(48), 55–76.

Aldridge, J., & Becker, S. (1999). Children as carers: the impact of parental illness and disability on children's caring roles. *Journal of Family Therapy, 21*(3), 303–320.

Banks, P., Cogan, N., Deeley, S., Hill, M., Riddell, S., & Tisdall, K. (2001). Seeing the invisible children and young people affected by disability. *Disability & Society, 16*(6), 797–814.

Banks, P., Cogan, N., Riddell, S., Hill, M., Deeley, S., & Tisdall, K. (2002). Does the covert nature of caring prohibit the development of effective services for young carers. *British Journal of Guidance & Counselling, 30*(3), 229–246.

Becker, S. (2007). Global perspectives on children's unpaid caregiving in the family: Research and policy on "young carers" in the UK, Australia, the USA and Sub-Saharan Africa. *Global Social Policy, 7*(1), 23–50.

Bolas, H., Van Wersch, A., & Flynn, D. (2007). The well-being of young people who care for a dependent relative: an interpretive phenomenological analysis. *Psychology and Health, 22*(7), 829–850.

Cree, V. E. (2003). Worries and problems of young carers: Issues for mental health. *Children and Family Social Work, 8*(4), 301–309.

Dearden, C., & Becker, S. (1998). *Young carers in the United Kingdom.* London: Carers National Association.

Dearden, C., & Becker, S. (2004). *Young carers in the UK: The 2004 report.* London: Carers UK.

Earley, L., & Cushway, D. J. (2002). The parentified child. *Clinical Child Psychology & Psychiatry, 7*(2), 163–178.

Frank, J., Tatum, C., & Tucker, S. (1999). *On small shoulders: Learning from the experiences of former young carers.* London: The Children's Society.

Kornblum, H., & Anderson, B. (1985). Parents with insulin dependent diabetes: Impact on family and child development. In S. Thurman (Ed.). *Children of handicapped parents: Research in clinical perspectives.* London: Academic Press.

Metzing-Blau, S., & Schnepp, W. (2008). Young carers in Germany: To live on as normal as possible—a grounded theory study. *BMC Nursing, 7*(1), 15–23.

Miles, M. B., & Huberman, A. M. (1984). *Qualitative data analysis: a sourcebook of new methods.* Newbury Park, CA: Sage.

Newman, T. (2002). "Young carers" and disabled parents: Time for a change of direction? *Disability & Society, 17*(6), 613–625.

Olsen, R. (1996). Young carers: Challenging the facts and politics of research into children and caring. *Disability & Society, 11*(1), 41–54.

Pakenham, K. I. (2009). Children who care for their parents: the impact of disability on young lives. In C. A. Marshall, E. Kendall, M. E. Banks, & R. M. S. Gover (Eds.). *Disability: insights from across fields and around the world* (Vol. 2). Westport, CT: Praeger Press.

Pakenham, K. I., & Bursnall, S. (2006). Relations between social support, appraisal and coping and both positive and negative outcomes for children of a parent with MS and comparisons with children of healthy parents. *Clinical Rehabilitation, 20*(8), 709–723.

Pakenham, K. I., Bursnall, S., Chiu, J., Cannon, T., & Okochi, M. (2006). The psychosocial impact of caregiving on young people who have a parent with an illness or disability: Comparisons between young caregivers and non-caregivers. *Rehabilitation Psychology, 51*(2), 113–126.

Pakenham, K. I., Chiu, J., Bursnall, S., & Cannon, T. (2007). Relations between social support, appraisal and coping and both positive and negative outcomes in young carers. *Journal of Health Psychology, 12*(1), 89–102.

Pakenham, K. I., & Cox, S. (2012). Test of a model of the effects of parental illness on youth and family functioning. *Health psychology 31*(5), 580–590.

Rolland, J. S. (1999). Parental Illness and disability: a family systems framework. *Journal of Family Therapy, 21*(3), 242–266.

Segal, J., & Simkins, J. (1993). *My mum needs me: Helping children with ill or disabled parents.* Hamondsworth: Penguin.

Shifren, K., & Kachorek, L. V. (2003). Does early caregiving matter? The effects on young caregivers' adult mental health.*International Journal of Behavioral Development, 27*(4), 338–346.

Worsham, N. L., Compass, B. E., & Sydney, E. Y. (1997).Children's coping with parental illness. In S. A. Wolchik, & I. N. Sandler (Eds.).*Handbook of Children's Coping: Linking Theory and Intervention* (pp. 195–213). New York: Plenum Press.

CHAPTER 7

Assisting Siblings When Their Brother or Sister Sustains Acquired Brain Injury

Samantha Bursnall

B rothers and sisters often share a life-long relationship. Because of the length and intensity of this relationship, they greatly influence one another's development, behaviors, personality, attitudes, and identity, independent of their genes or parental influences (Cicirelli, 1995). Because siblings are such a large part of each other's lives, it is not surprising that when one sustains an acquired brain injury (ABI), the other siblings can be greatly affected— sometimes for many years following the injury or illness.

This chapter tells a story based on the experiences of 24 young Australians whose brother or sister sustained an ABI. It gives an understanding of the difficulties and experiences siblings face and identifies ways to assist them to cope. Although the onset of a life-changing event, such as a child's ABI, is different for every individual, there are some common experiences that siblings are likely to feel. The young people who shared their experiences here have provided some important information and advice for parents and other siblings who may find themselves in a similar situation in the future. Understanding the experiences of siblings is an important first step in assisting them to cope.

The Sibling Story

Having a brother or sister acquire a brain injury can be devastating for a young person. The siblings who shared their stories described it as a life-changing event affecting their entire family. The event caused turmoil, trauma, confusion, and changes that had lasting consequences. One teenage girl shared, ". . . the whole situation . . . sort of turned our lives upside down . . ." Another young person recalled that, "the whole family just changed automatically. It was a really weird and quick change. . . ." The effects of these changes are often ongoing as described by one boy who talked about the impact of his brother's brain injury several years after the injury: "When it first happened it was very hard, sometimes it's still very hard. . . . That still is a big thing in my life."

Emergency, Intensive Care, and Hospital

When a child is first injured and requires a lot of medical care and attention, it can be a particularly stressful time for siblings because it is fuelled by a range of emotions. It is important to remember, however, that although these experiences are most prominent in the first few months of a young person's injury, their impact can be felt for many years after the event.

The Screaming Brakes

Siblings might be present when their brother or sister sustains their injury or becomes ill. Some described witnessing their brother or sister sustain the injury as a traumatic, terrifying, frightening, confusing, and a surreal experience that they were able to recall vividly years after the injury. Although it differed in degree, those who witnessed their brother or sister's injury said they still experienced visual or auditory memories of the accident many years later. Many described experiencing intrusive thoughts, flashbacks, and dreams about the incident. Although most of these siblings said that with time they thought and dreamt about the event less often, its impact still appeared to be long-lived. One boy described how seven years after his brother's ABI he still experienced flashbacks: "It was scary, daunting, it still comes back and you still think about it and you still feel it . . . The accident comes back all the time."

"The Accident Was All Because of Me"

Some siblings blamed themselves for their brother or sister's ABI, despite having no control over what happened. Some young people thought that if only they had done one thing differently, the injury would not have occurred, especially those who were nearby when the accident happened. They believed that if they were doing something wrong, such as fighting or arguing with their brother or sister before the injury occurred, the injury was their punishment for those behaviors. As one 11-year-old girl recalled, "I don't really like saying this but on the afternoon of the accident my sister wasn't doing as she was told . . . so I gave her a little bit of a smack and that's the reason why I blame myself a bit—if I hadn't smacked her, this wouldn't have happened. Because you know this was my pay back for hitting her . . . like inside I was feeling guilty."

The feeling of self-blame may not diminish for a long time as indicated by one boy who witnessed his brother fall several years previously: "I still tend to blame myself, it's silly but you know I don't do it as much anymore, but I used to all the time. People try to tell me that it's not my fault but I don't listen to it. Like I don't really think it is, I sort of do and sort of don't. Mum and dad said that it was an accident." Some siblings felt so bad they even wished that it had been themselves who were injured, like one teenage girl who said, "I started to think it was all my fault and then I remember I kept thinking I wish it had been me."

Taking responsibility and feeling guilt is sometimes referred to as survivor guilt (Lemberger, 1995). Parents and siblings may blame themselves because they perceive that they could have done something differently to have prevented the injury from occurring. People often blame themselves as a form of punishment—paying the penance for being healthy and well (Lemberger, 1995). They may also unconsciously believe that if they take responsibility this time, then they can control the future and prevent it from happening again. Survivor guilt may also be accompanied by other feelings like gratitude and relief, further increasing feelings of guilt. Although these reactions are common, it is important to seek some help to resolve these feelings.

"Is This My Bother?"

Seeing their brother or sister in the emergency room, the intensive care unit (ICU) or the hospital ward was described as shocking, scary, and confusing. Siblings were often overwhelmed at seeing the medical equipment attached to their brother or sister and could not understand why he or she was unconscious and unresponsive. They realized the seriousness of their sibling's condition but felt helpless to do anything about it. One boy said his brother "looked white and had all the tubes coming out of every crevice of his body." Another said, "When they took me down to see him in intensive care, I just started crying and I just broke down in front of him. Just seeing him with all those tubes in him . . . I woke up a bit and thought . . . I hope he gets out." The siblings who told their stories said they were confused about what a coma was and what it meant for their sibling: "I had never really seen anyone else who had gone into a coma and I had no idea what happened. . . . I was just really, really, really scared. It was very emotional and I felt really sad and I was crying a lot."

Witnessing their brother or sister in hospital with bandages and tubes around their body also triggered fears of death. Confronting the possible death of a family member, often for the first time, was overwhelming and frightening. Seeing their family member so close to death was described by one teenage girl as "really horrible, it was really scary . . . it was like, you know when you are on a swing and you stomach just goes—that sort of feeling. As soon as I saw him I thought there's no way he is going to come out of here."

"You Don't Know What to Feel... It's Real Turmoil Inside"

Not surprisingly, the siblings who told their stories said that they felt a great deal of anxiety and mixed emotions. One boy who was 15 when his sister had a car accident said, ". . . first week when she was in intensive care I was upset heaps. I couldn't even sleep or anything, I was that worried" and another girl agreed, "I was so worried about my sick brother, and I was worried about mum and dad."

Much of the worry reported by siblings was related to the unknown future outcomes of their brother's or sister's health and whether they would survive. Although many were told that if their brothers or sisters lived they would have brain damage, most did not understand what this meant. One boy recalled his fear of the unknown, "I was worried about her heaps . . . What she was going to turn out like after it—Did she have brain damage? Or, what's going to happen?" These concerns also turned to questions about their future relationship with their injured brother or sister. "Is she going to be the same with me? 'Cause . . . me and her were really close . . . I would talk to her about anything, I was mainly worried about how she would turn out after it." Another teenager described having similar concerns, "I thought about how he is going to turn out in the future, if he will ever be able to talk properly again?"

In addition to feeling intense worry, some young people also experienced emotional turmoil, such as feeling shock, numbness, isolation, and sadness. Others felt moody, depressed, and frustrated about the situation, like one teenager who said he physically took out his frustration and anger on his peers: "I was pretty annoyed with the world so my friend asked me not to beat the hell out of anyone in the football game. I was thinking about other things rather than thinking about the game I was playing." One teenage girl said that "everyone's emotions are going a bit whacked, sort of like shock, like hitting a brick wall . . . I just wanted to say—stop please!" Many young people in this situation also said that it was common for them to have difficulty concentrating at school and lost interest in extracurricular activities and friends: "It just made my (school grades) go down because I couldn't concentrate and that, and I didn't have time for my friends, and even my sport went down the tube. I couldn't concentrate on the ground, I used to (stop playing sport) sometimes, just not interested."

Even adults, who were children or teenagers when their brother or sister sustained their injury, said they remembered this time and how they felt. One adult said, "You just feel so—devastated. You feel so in turmoil . . . you don't know what to feel. 'Cause you don't really know what's happened. . . . You don't know what to feel sad about, but everyone's feeling so sad, and stressed, so, you think you have to too. So it's like it's real turmoil inside . . . "

Life as these young people and their families had always known it was put on hold while the entire family focused their energy on the child with the ABI. One teenage boy said that while his sister was in hospital he "didn't want to do anything, didn't want to go out. I was just at the hospital every day." Another said, "Try and get my mind off it—that was a very hard task because I was thinking about it constantly."

"I Never Used to Get to Spend Much Time with My Parents"

Also difficult for siblings was the amount of time they spent without their parents, especially in the beginning when their brother or sister is in hospital. This left siblings to look after themselves or be looked after by friends or relatives. When asked about the impact of this time, stories commonly echoed experiences such as ". . . My parents were worried and they were always at the hospital . . . dad usually stayed the night there and mum would come home at night. For about three months friends gave us dinners because our parents weren't home to cook."

When asked about how they felt about not seeing their parents as much, many of the siblings agreed: ". . . it sort of got me jealous a bit when Mum and Dad were never home for us. I had to do all my assignments without her . . . but I got there eventually." Others described feeling left out: ". . . When she first came out of hospital I was a bit jealous. My parents were still paying attention to me, but it just felt different. It was Betty this and Betty that, and it should have been." Even older siblings who understood the loss of attention said they still felt jealous and unsupported. Siblings in this situation described feeling lonely, like one boy who said, "It was just mainly the first one or two years that I was lonely because I never used to see Mum and Dad much. It's alright now, though, I see them a lot." Some siblings felt unacknowledged. "I remember feeling left out when people would ring me for information, like relatives and friends . . . and they would go 'How's your Mum, how's your brother (with ABI)?' . . . and I was thinking 'what about Fred (other well sibling) and I'? . . . not Mum and Dad so much . . . but feeling left out that other people didn't consider us."

The loss of parent's time and attention often continued even when their sibling came home from hospital, in that their parents' time, energy, and resources continued to be allocated to the child with ABI. For example, siblings noticed that more time was given to the injured child, they received more gifts, and their wrongful behavior was more likely to be overlooked. Some siblings even perceived their parents to be closer to their brother or sister since the injury.

Even though they felt lonely, left out, or jealous, they still understood the difficult position their parents were in and the worry they were expressing. Siblings understood and accepted their parents need to be at the hospital or at rehabilitation, because ultimately their brother or sister needed the extra time. One young girl said, "Just like try to understand it, that they are busy and everything, your Mum and Dad, they need to look after him."

"Trying to Hide It So Your Parents Don't Worry"

One of the experiences siblings found most difficult was seeing their parents upset and distressed, especially when their brother or sister was in hospital and for some time after. Parents are the people to whom children turn for comfort when they experience difficult times, however siblings said that seeing their parents in this situation made them reluctant to talk to them about how they were feeling in case they upset them even more. Instead, the siblings attempted to put on a brave face and act in control. They wanted to be perceived, especially by their parents, to be coping well and this was their way of helping the family in a time of turmoil. This strategy however, will likely affect the level of support they receive and inadvertently increase their isolation and loneliness. Despite these feelings, the siblings said it was still their preference to talk to their parents about their thoughts/feelings, and those who actually did so said they felt much better.

Return Home, Rehabilitation, and Onward

The experience of siblings, particularly when their brother or sister was first injured showed that siblings are affected in myriad ways. In addition, to some of the life changes and traumatic experiences described above, siblings also had to adjust to challenges when their brother or sister returned home. They had to adjust to new routines and to changes in their brother or sister who appeared to be just like a different person—physically, emotionally, and/or psychologically.

"Far out! She's Not the Same!"

Many siblings only noticed the full impact of the changes when their brother or sister returned home. This time caused confusion for siblings whose brother or sister looked the same as prior to the injury, but did not behave in the same way: "At the start I . . . was expecting her to be normal. Like I would stir her like I normally do, and she couldn't take it and that's when we used to start fighting."

The siblings had to adjust to many physical, emotional, behavioral, and personality changes in their brother or sister, which had a profound impact on their relationship. They described being confused about the changes, unprepared for them, and unable to deal with them. For many it was like getting to know a familiar stranger. Comments like, "My brother . . . is not himself, he's had a total like different personality change" were common. The most disturbing changes were those related to a sense of unpredictability and fragility. The hardest change to adjust to seemed to be the erratic, unpredictable, and variable behavior (including, violence or risk-taking), which siblings found confusing and difficult to understand as well as stressful and frustrating. On the other hand, siblings also saw their brother or sister as being more fragile since their injury: "When you see your brother so close to death, it makes it very real the possibility that you could see them there again."

Some adults, who were children when their brother or sister had their injury, said that the changes in their brother or sister required gradual adjustment and that these changes impacted on their lives daily for many years following the injury: "After the accident, straight away, you know it's something bad. You just don't understand that he is not going to be the same . . . I never sobbed about it then. Never. Not until I got a bit older and thought, you know, 'Oh boy, this is pretty ordinary'. It keeps impacting every day. It's been an experience . . . growing up with my brother the way he is."

Siblings expressed a deep sense of loss as a result of the changes in the sibling with ABI. They grieved for the loss of interactions, advice, and relationship they previously had with their brother or sister. They also grieved for the person they had lost and the person they could have been. The loss siblings felt was described as constant and everlasting.

"I Protect Him Because I Don't Want to Have to Go through That Again"

The changes in the child with ABI, such as their unpredictability and fragility, led many siblings to feel continuous worry. Siblings constantly thought about their sibling's safety, their health outcomes, and their future. They also felt concerned when their brother or sister displayed unusual behaviors and wondered what this meant for their health. One sibling said, "I just get worried that he may die . . . And, I get worried about Mum and Dad having to look after him when he is sick because it is a stress."

As a result of the changes and consequent perceived vulnerability to recurring injury or death, siblings became very protective. Their protective tendencies included keeping a watchful eye on their brother or sister, monitoring their activities, helping them with rehabilitation, and protecting them from danger in public or from bullies in the schoolyard. For example, one teenage boy said "now, I have got to be on the watch . . . I just look after him, watch what he does . . . It's all pretty much the way I feel just trying to protect him, because I don't want to have to go through that again." They also said that they did not physically fight back as much as they used to because they did not want to hurt their brother or sister any further. As one young boy described, "I would never get physical with him if he annoyed me because I didn't want to hurt him anymore than he already has been."

As a result of all these changes, siblings found they played a different role with their brother or sister with ABI. For example, those who were younger became the older sibling and in some cases, more like a parent. One boy who was younger than his brother said, "Like I am the big brother sort of thing now."

"I Would Just Feel Guilty about Everything"

As well as the mix of emotions described above, siblings expressed a deep sense of sorrow for their brother or sister after their brain injury and for their resulting disabilities and illness. They felt sorrow that their brother or sister had to continually take medicine, and that they had lost the friends, jobs, and activities they were involved in before. As a result, siblings expressed feelings of guilt because their siblings could no longer do the things that they themselves could still do. One 10-year-old girl said, "I wish he didn't have this injury because then he could do all this fun stuff and everything. He could like go on rides and everything at the show . . . I feel sorry because he can't come with me because he always wants to go on rides . . . I wish he didn't have this injury."

Siblings also became frustrated, stressed, angry, and embarrassed about their brothers' or sisters' behavior at times. One girl said, "It is very stressful sometimes . . . sometimes you can just sort of like go and scream!" And, "he acts a bit inappropriately in public . . . it's a bit embarrassing." Some siblings found it frustrating at times because they missed out on doing things and going to places because their brother or sister was unable to go or because their parents were busy doing other things for their brother or sister. At the same time, however, siblings also described feeling guilty and ashamed for being embarrassed, frustrated, or angry. They said they felt guilty because they knew their brother or sister could not help their situation and because of the strong bond and love they had for them: "I felt so guilty. Every time I did something or started enjoying myself I would start thinking I can't do this, I can't have fun. I would just feel guilty about everything—and then later wanting to do things like go camping and asking to go and then feeling guilty because we couldn't go, or because I had even bothered asking . . . I still feel like my brother never got to do this and that and Mum and Dad are at home working so hard looking after him and I am here."

Overall, siblings experienced a mix of emotions, including anger, jealousy, loss, guilt, fear, anxiety, frustration, and sorrow. They often bottled up their feelings and tried to accept the situation. Some resisted the changes whereas others withdrew from the situation, went for a walk, played sport, or listened to music.

"It Just Makes You Realize What You've Still Got"

The siblings described many personal changes as a result of having a brother or sister with ABI. They described an increased understanding of disability and more tolerance of differences between people. They also said they were more patient in general as a result of having to be more patient with their sibling, as well as more independent. They also described themselves as being more responsible and mature, and less likely to take risks with dangerous activities. One teenage boy said, "I just got more responsible with things, with heaps of different things." Others said they felt that their sibling's injury provided them with the opportunity for personal growth and many positive experiences. As one teenager said, "There have been sacrifices, but I don't look at it as a losing experience, I see that I have gained an experience." Many siblings also said that since their brother or sister was injured, they had developed an increased appreciation of life: "It just makes you realize what you've still got, I mean you don't know how much you miss something until it is gone. I am still the same. Exactly the same, it's just that I like my brother, you know, I love him but you only say that when you are about to die or something . . . Like we still cared about each other but we never showed it before the injury."

Strategies for Assisting Siblings

The type of support given to siblings will often depend on such things as the age of the sibling, their friendship networks, familial support, and their living environment. As described so far, however, there are many complex processes impacting on how young people react to their brothers' or sisters' brain injury. It is important to remember that ABI impacts on every individual and every family member differently. Therefore, when assisting siblings, one must keep in mind that each person should be listened to carefully and their individual experiences and needs assessed. The young people who told their stories made some recommendations about what helped them to cope or what support they would have liked to have had to be able to cope better. These tips may be useful to others in future.

Encourage Communication

Given that siblings often witnessed their sibling's injury, interventions should include debriefing, information, inclusion, communication, and validation. Debriefing helps people to process their thoughts, beliefs, and feelings about an event, particularly when they have witnessed something traumatic. Often a staff member at the hospital arranged for someone experienced to talk to siblings about their fears, guilt, anxieties, and concerns, as in the case with one teenage boy who said, "She (the counselor) would make me feel better and stuff like that. She explained to me what actually happened to his brain. And, like how, if you injure your right part, your left part of your body goes down and vice-versa. She was pretty nice. Like I told her a lot and she was pretty good and made me feel a lot better." Talking to family and close friends also helped siblings enormously. Even though it may seem daunting, talking helps young people to get things off their chest and access appropriate support.

It may be that siblings feel the need to talk about their experience at length, for some time after the accident, as the sibling experience changes. Advice from one 16-year-old boy reflected what many other siblings said, "You have to talk about it otherwise you just sit there and don't want to talk about it. . . . You let it out and you let your feelings out, and you can tell someone and then you understand it. You feel better once you get it out."

It was crucial that schools were informed about the impact of an ABI on family members. Encouraging teachers to offer siblings' support and perhaps lessening their workloads, particularly when their brother or sister is first injured, is likely to facilitate them through the initial period of change and transition thereafter.

Appropriate Information: Preparation and Inclusion

Most siblings wished for as much information as possible about their sibling's brain injury. They wanted this information in age-appropriate language and to be told the truth. Information is usually available in booklets and brochures given out at hospitals or at various nonprofit organizations. However, little of this information is child-friendly. Nurses and doctors also often help by providing information to siblings.

It is important to prepare siblings for the first time they see their brother or sister in hospital, especially in terms of the medical equipment. Siblings wanted to be kept in the loop of communication, particularly those who were older. Some younger siblings said they would have preferred information to come from their parents, although as long as they understood it, they did not mind where it came from. Some siblings even liked to be involved in their sibling's recovery and rehabilitation.

Overall, siblings wanted to be given a choice. However, some of the younger siblings were pleased that they had only received limited information because more details about the injury may have upset them further. In addition, all siblings said it was important that they were sufficiently prepared for what to expect when their brother or sister returned home, including how the ABI may affect their behavior and how to handle the changes and challenges. Above all, they wanted the people around them to remain hopeful and positive.

Normalize and Validate Feelings

It was very important for siblings to know that their feelings, such as those discussed in this chapter, were normal and common. It was also important to encourage siblings to talk about their concerns and find someone who would listen to them. Educating and sensitizing parents to the experiences and needs of siblings was also essential, given the tendency of siblings to repress their feelings. Parents should set up an environment which shows that talking about feelings is acceptable. Those who do not wish to talk to anyone should be encouraged to write down their feelings through letters, journals, diaries, blogs, or online support forums. As one boy said, he had "a lot of deep conversations with mum that helped a lot with accepting the situation for what it was." Communication during the initial stages of the recovery process is imperative, because initial coping patterns often appear to remain dominant throughout the recovery process (Bursnall, 2003).

Acknowledge Siblings' Contributions

It is also important that the difficulties and sacrifices siblings make when their brother or sister sustains an injury are acknowledged. Many siblings put on a brave face and attempt to be strong for the entire family, sometimes for years after the injury. No matter how unaffected siblings may appear, it is important that their contributions, trials, and achievements are recognized. Some siblings said that what helped them to get through the tough times was knowing that the sacrifices they made and the things they gave up for their brother or sister were noticed by their parents and acknowledged. They also said that acknowledgment of the extra responsibilities they took on, especially the less obvious ones, helped them cope: "My teacher always says what a good job I did looking after the house and my other siblings. It was hard sometimes. It helps to know that all you do is appreciated. That makes it so much easier to keep going . . . My Mom used to come home and tell me that I am doing a good job and everything, so that was good because it gave me that boost to keep going."

Acknowledging the unique difficulties siblings experience, the hard work and responsibilities they may acquire, the patience and understanding they need, as well as the things they miss out on, can go a long way to supporting siblings. It is also important that siblings are not expected to care for their brother or sister with ABI constantly. Siblings sometimes need time to themselves or to be with their friends alone.

Time-out with Parents and Respite

Even though it is often difficult for parents to arrange time out, siblings said that spending special time alone with parents helped them to feel better. It also helped when someone, especially their parents, clearly explained to them that they were still special. Younger children sometimes display changes in their behavior in response to the perceived unfairness or inequity in the changed family environment. Explaining the change to them in clear language may help them manage the situation better. Encouraging siblings to go out with friends on their own and to continue their sport, activities, school, hobbies, and interests is crucial to maintain normality and return to stability and routine as soon as possible. One sibling said, "After two weeks I went back to school. I had other things to think about, like formulas for Physics and stuff and I just, I tried to think about other things, I just really put an effort into thinking about other things."

Sharing Similar Experiences

Some siblings gained enormous support from hearing the stories of other siblings in a similar situation. Hearing such stories let them know what others went through and how they coped, which helped them to feel supported and understood: "You wouldn't be able to understand until it happened to you. Just knowing that someone else is in a similar situation helps . . . you help each other . . . You talk and you give advice . . . share a bit of information and give a different way to handle things."

Other strategies to support siblings come in the form of DVDs that capture the sibling experience (Bursnall, 2005; Siblings Australia, 2012) and internet groups, where siblings (children or adults) with special needs can talk online and share their experiences. Encouraging parents and siblings to view such media together may assist in opening the channels for communication.

Conclusion

It has been shown that life after ABI can present many changes, challenges, and learning experiences for all of those affected. Like all family members, siblings are also affected in a myriad of ways. The stories shared by the siblings in this chapter reflected the strength, resilience, patience, and maturity in managing the life change presented to them when their playmate, confidante, and life's companion was struck with an ABI. Siblings mostly cope extraordinarily well, however, they may also experience many underlying fears, anxieties, feelings, thoughts, and concerns that they find hard to understand and comprehend. These experiences can be somewhat alleviated when they are provided with support, compassion, understanding, and acknowledgment.

Acknowledgments

Special thanks to the siblings who took part in this study, sharing their experiences to assist others in a similar situation. This chapter is based on research funded by the Financial Markets Foundation for Children and a smaller version appeared in a consumer publication produced by the Brain Injury Association of Queensland.

References

Bursnall, S. (2003). *Regaining equilibrium: Understanding the process of sibling adjustment to paediatric acquired brain injury.* Unpublished manuscript, Department of Health and Human Services, Griffith University, Brisbane, Queensland, Australia.

Bursnall, S. (2005). *Out of the shadows: Understanding the experience of siblings following their brother or sister's acquired brain injury* [DVD]. Bendigo, Victoria: Video Education Australasia.

Cicirelli, V. G. (1995). *Sibling relationships across the life span.* New York: Plenum Press.

Lemberger, J. (1995). *A global perspective on working with Holocaust survivors and the second generation.* Jerusalem: JDC-Brookdale Institute of Gerontology and Human Development in cooperation with the World Council of Jewish Communal Service.

Siblings Australia Inc. & Turner, S. (2012). *Stronger siblings: Support for brothers and sisters of children with disability* [DVD]. Adelaide, South Australia: Siblings Australia Inc.

PART 3

SYSTEMS FOR HEALING: BUILDING A BETTER SERVICE SYSTEM FOR TRAUMATIC BRAIN INJURY

Heidi Muenchberger

Brain injury is a lifelong event, but disability and secondary health conditions related to brain injury (i.e., social and psychological impact) can be mitigated and even avoided. Nine out of ten people require rehabilitation support following discharge from the health system (AIHW, 2007), but often must fend for themselves or rely on family and friends for this support in the short-term. Once medically stable, individuals living with brain injury may no longer receive any formal rehabilitation. However, significant social, emotional, and behavioral dysfunction can emerge over time, leading to secondary disabilities (e.g., subsequent traumatic brain injuries, mental illness, and drug dependence), overdependence on primary health services and readmission to hospital. This situation is preventable if a strong service delivery system is established in the first instance. This section of the book highlights the components of a strong service delivery system, which include group-based support programs (incorporating meta-cognitive skills development using real-life therapeutic settings), peer feedback as a central agent of change and motivation, intensive staff commitment, multidisciplinary assessment, and goal-setting for the future.

During 2009 and 2010, I undertook an international Churchill Fellowship to investigate the pathways of brain injury recovery (see Muenchberger, 2010). Findings from this fellowship confirmed the benefits of maintaining well-being following brain injury, including the need for a focus on positive activity and health promotion strategies. Simple strategies such as maintaining a healthy diet, exercise, and relaxation had a sustainable effect over time, but were often neglected. In addition, the client–practitioner relationship and importance of social networks within the community were key facilitators of progress over the long-term. The chapters in this section emerged from this fellowship and represented some of the most innovative models that had been implemented around the world. Each of the approaches contained in this section of the book emphasize the capacity of individuals with brain injury to change and grow over time. However, they also acknowledge that without responsive service systems and relationship-focused professionals, change may go unnoticed, and growth may be hindered.

People with brain injury are more likely than many other people with disabilities to require assistance from multiple services, with the greatest demand being for community support, case management, and psychosocial support (AIHW, 2007). Studies have confirmed that even up to 25 years postinjury, the main sources of disability following brain injury are those related to mental health and behavioral symptoms (Hoofinen, Gilboa, Vakil, & Donovick, 2003). Over 90 percent of people with brain injury receive subacute inpatient rehabilitation for periods of greater than 50 days, but only 5.6 percent receive any psychological intervention during their rehabilitation (AIHW, 2007). Delays in treatment are often associated with severe behavioral or psychiatric problems and represent a significant cost to the health system.

Importantly, improvements in physical, psychological, and social health have been noted over the long-term (up to 20 years postinjury), indicating that secondary prevention efforts are as important as primary care, but also highlighting the importance of long-term follow up and treatment. Interventions designed to provide innovative psychological support and understanding are gathering broader recognition, and emphasis is increasingly being focused on optimization therapies (i.e., making the most of everything you have) rather than deficit-reduction approaches.

Although individual treatments can facilitate important outcomes, the capacity of the health professionals and services to communicate and coordinate supports over time and location is critical. People living with brain injury may miss out on valuable services due to the fragmentation and lack of coordination between rehabilitation services. Given the diverse multidisciplinary input over the brain injury rehabilitation trajectory, communication between services becomes even more vital. Limited access to timely and appropriate psychosocial or behavioral rehabilitation services at the beginning of the care trajectory may contribute to increased problems at a later date, resulting in repeat presentations to primary care services and frequent use of community mental health facilities. For observers in this field, it could be concluded that successful long-term outcomes might reflect a case of good luck rather than deliberate planning (see Muenchberger, Kendall, & Collings, 2011 for detailed discussion).

Our recent research into the meaning of holistic brain injury rehabilitation (Wright & Muenchberger, 2011) has indicated that holistic rehabilitation is the result of a combined effect of individual practitioner skills, system capacity to coordinate services, and quality standards. It seems unreasonable to expect any individual health professional to properly deliver holistic rehabilitation within their scope of practice. Holistic rehabilitation demands a combined response from multidisciplinary teams and a whole-of-system response (including quality referral pathways).

The chapters within this section of the book discuss the need for an inclusive or holistic focus on the physical, psychological, functional, and social environment in order to deal with the complexity of brain injury. They discuss the complexity created by the continued prevalence of pathogenesis and our reticence to examine models of flourishing and mental well-being in brain injury. They describe how the cultural and philosophical underpinnings of traditional *deficit* approaches are difficult to shift, but offer viable alternatives that have been demonstrated in applied settings across multiple countries. These chapters discuss the importance of the clinical exchange whereby the relationship established between the health professional and client remains core to the therapeutic endeavor and is a precondition for any positive outcome. They focus on the need to provide opportunities for people with brain injuries and to recognize the complexity of the circumstances within which they operate.

With a global trend toward reduced lengths of hospital stay and earlier discharge to community-based rehabilitation services, coordination and cooperation between hospital and community services and health practitioners becomes more important (Cope, Mayer, & Cervelli, 2007). In this context, we need to move toward a responsive, not reactive, system. In order to deliver the best rehabilitation, the service system, the community, consumers, researchers, and health professionals must have the capacity to deliver improved outcomes. Without building capacity across a number of sectors, brain injury services will continue to be reactive and, by necessity, crisis motivated.

References

Australian Institute of Health and Welfare (AIHW) (2007). *Disability in Australia: Acquired brain injury in Australia*. AIHW Bulletin 55. Canberra, Australian Capital Territory: Australia.

Cope, N., Mayer, N., & Cervelli, L. (2005). Development of systems of care for persons with traumatic brain injury. *Journal of Head Trauma Rehabilitation, 20*(2), 128–142.

Hoofinen, D., Gilboa, A., Vakil, E., & Donovick, P. (2003). Traumatic brain injury (TBI) 10–20 years later: a comprehensive outcome study of psychiatric symptomatology, cognitive abilities and psychosocial functioning. *Brain Injury, 15*(3), 189–209.

Muenchberger, H. (2010). Churchill Report. The Churchill Trust. DOI http://www.churchilltrust.com.au/fellows/detail/3368/

Muenchberger, H., Kendall, E., & Collings, C. (2011). Beyond crisis care in brain injury: a conversation worth having. *Journal of Primary Care and Community Health, 2*(1), 60–64.

Wright, C., & Muenchberger, M. (2011). *Holistic practice in traumatic brain injury rehabilitation: Perspectives of health practitioners* (Honours dissertation, Griffith University, 2011).

SEWING

Grab your limbs we need a needle, I'll sew you back together, with
thread—

Stars slice raw the silver flesh of un-seamed past. I'll sew your
wounds to scares, flesh leaking crimson no more.

It's okay. I know your name. I'll use a thimble

Unravelling under a willow, Grab a pillow, Lay perfectly still, I have
a seam ripper if the scars won't heal

Quilted skin, inseams a mystery—we all look pristine.

Bring you left hand—or is it lost? It may not write for you, but you
want it, don't you?

I'll stitch you back together. Stuff you with goose down feathers.

Howl at the moon and I'll howl too. Piercing your skin with silver
moonlight thread

Are you dead? Not me—perfectly aware we could be zombies.

Ripped and shredded,

Even poor boys go to heaven

Sifting through dirt, grab you head—I'll bolt that on too, I'll stitch
you to look brand new.

Tie off loose ends. Only the sun makes the night sky seam surreal.

Eyes watching. Don't they have limbs need sewing?

Unravelling mess, preying eyes look at my blood stained dress.

We are mending your arm when we find a needle and thread

Ripped, stitched, warren, torn, bleached, eventually dyed, fabric of
time is all mine.

I could live in a tree, weeds, remarkably even under the sea, possibly the city too, but not without you.

We have all your limbs . . .

I have a needle!

With a thimble you can howl . . .

and I will weave in and out.

Erica Anderson

CHAPTER 8

Understanding Mental Health Outcomes following Traumatic Brain Injury

Maria Hennessy

When considering mental health outcomes for traumatic brain injury (TBI) survivors, there is a tendency to view these from a traditional medical model that monitors levels of symptom distress and the presence or absence of psychopathology. This chapter contends that recovery and outcomes following a TBI need to be reconsidered using a dual-factor model of mental health that includes both mental illness and mental well-being. The extant body of research that has examined mental illness following TBI suggests that individuals are at increased risk for the development of a range of depression and anxiety disorders. Of concern is an apparent increase, not decrease, in the development of mental illness over time. It is difficult to draw firm conclusions from the aforesaid literature about the diagnosis, incidence, prevalence, risk factors, and temporal course of mental illness following a TBI due to a number of common methodological concerns. Research has not investigated mental well-being to any significant degree following TBI. Prospective longitudinal outcome studies are required that describe the natural progression of mental well-being and mental illness following a TBI. A focus on positive mental health and consumer-defined recovery should inform the development and integration of innovative health services to support the recovery of individuals following a TBI.

What Is Mental Health?

Our concepts and understanding of mental health are dynamic and evolving. For the majority of individuals, both lay people and health professionals, mental health is synonymous with mental illness. The assessment, treatment, and management of mental health problems are firmly rooted in a pathogenic tradition that views health as the absence of disease and disability (Keyes, 2007). From this traditional medical perspective, mental health is assumed to represent a single unipolar dimension with mental illness at one end of a spectrum and mental health at the other (Keyes, 2005). Mental health outcomes within public mental health services are still primarily conceptualized from within a medical model with its focus on the management of psychopathology, levels of symptom distress, number of acute hospitalizations, and medication compliance (Andresen, Caputi, & Oades, 2010; Antaramian, Huebner, Hill, & Valois, 2010).

However, health in general has long been regarded as a complete state that includes coexisting domains of positive well-being and illness (Gurin, Veroff, & Feld, 1960). Jahoda (1958) described a framework for positive mental health that contained six components namely acceptance of oneself, growth/development/becoming, integration of personality, autonomy, accurate perception of reality, and environmental mastery. Five decades later, the World Health Organization (WHO) (1948) defined mental health as a complete state of well-being where the individual can cope with the normal stresses of life, work productively,

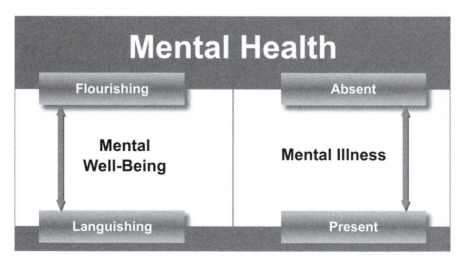

Figure 8.1 The dual-factor model of mental health, mental well-being, and mental illness.

and contribute to his or her community. There is a growing consensus that mental health should be considered a holistic state that includes the two coexisting but independent factors of mental illness and mental well-being (Manderscheid et al., 2010). Mental well-being and mental illness can therefore be conceptualized as the dual factors that underlie mental health (see Figure 8.1).

Understanding Mental Illness

We understand the term mental illness far better than we do mental well-being. Mental illness refers to the spectrum of diagnosable psycho-pathological states that interfere with an individual's emotional, social, and cognitive abilities. The assessment, understanding, and treatment of mental illness have been the primary focus of clinical psychology and psychiatry since the mid-1940s. Considerable progress has been made in this regard. For instance, we are able to reliably measure symptoms of the most common mental illnesses such as depression, anxiety, and schizo-phrenia; utilize evidence-based psychological and pharmacological treat-ments to relieve symptom distress; and gain an understanding of the complex interplay between genetics and environmental stressors that con-tribute to the expression and maintenance of mental illness (Duckworth, Steen, & Seligman, 2005). However, such approaches continue to regard mental health as the absence of psychopathology (Keyes, 2007). A di-chotomous focus on the negative or illness components of mental health minimizes if not negates the importance of positive emotions as a sepa-rate psychological process, mediated by different neural substrates, and potentially with an evolutionary function that is distinct from negative emotions (Duckworth et al., 2005; Fredrickson, 2003). As Duckworth et al. (2005) state, ". . . the mere relief of suffering does not lead to well-being; it only removes one of the barriers to well-being. Well-being is a process over and above the absence of depression, anxiety, and anger" (p. 234).

Mental Illness following Traumatic Brain Injury

Despite the large numbers of individuals who sustain a TBI each year, we still have a limited understanding of who develops a mental illness following a TBI, and what the critical periods for development are. The natural course of recovery is still unclear although it appears that the first year postinjury is critical, and that for some individuals, TBI may cause decades-long vulnerability to psychiatric illness (Gould, Ponsford, Johnston, & Schonberger, 2011; Hoofien, Gilboa, Vakil, & Donovick, 2001). The purpose of the following section is to highlight selected find-ings that have implications for clinical practice and service delivery. The interested reader is referred to Kim et al. (2007) and Rogers and Read (2007) for more detailed reviews of specific psychiatric disorders following TBI.

Prior to considering the literature noted below, it is important to highlight a number of common methodological concerns that make it difficult to draw firm conclusions about the diagnosis, incidence, prevalence, risk factors, and temporal course of mental illness following a TBI. These are summarized in Table 8.1. From a clinical perspective, the different methods used for the diagnosis of psychiatric disorders are particularly problematic.

Table 8.1 Common methodological concerns in the literature investigating mental illness following traumatic brain injury

Methodological Concern	Example
Different methods used for psychiatric diagnoses	Comprehensive structured clinical interviews versus brief symptom checklists Current diagnoses only are often recorded, not those that have resolved post-TBI
Differences in injury severity	Majority of literature based on moderate to severe TBI Often heterogeneous mild, moderate and severe TBI groups
Variable times since injury	Ranging from 3 months to 30 years
Different sampling methods	Randomized versus self-selected
Limited length of time for follow-up	Majority focuses on the first year post-TBI
Different sampling settings	Inpatient rehabilitation, community
Use of cross-sectional samples	Do not enable determination of the actual change over time for the individual Potential for cohort effects
Use of retrospective reporting	Reliability of self-report up to a decade postinjury
Lack of preinjury information	Absent versus comprehensive structured clinical interviews
Selection of assessment instruments	Often have undemonstrated reliability and validity with a TBI population
Limited cross-cultural information	Majority of research conducted in westernized countries such as United States, United Kingdom, Canada, and Australia
Limited geographic information	Role of geography in recovery (e.g., urban versus rural) is often neglected.

The use of a structured clinical interview, clinical screen, or symptom checklist will produce varying psychiatric profiles between assessors and make it difficult to reliably determine actual levels of mental illness post-TBI. The other significant methodological issue is time, in terms of both time since injury, and the predominance of cross-sectional samples. It is difficult to describe the natural course of recovery following TBI when time samples vary from months to decades postinjury, and very few studies are prospective in design. It is with these cautions in mind that the following literature is considered.

Individuals with a TBI are more likely to experience a mental illness compared to the general population, with consistently elevated incidence and prevalence rates for psychiatric disorders such as depression (e.g., major depressive disorder, depression not otherwise specified) and anxiety (e.g., posttraumatic stress disorder, generalized anxiety disorder, panic disorder, obsessive-compulsive disorder) (Bombardier et al., 2010; Gould et al., 2011; Kim et al., 2007). Estimated prevalence of depressive disorders following TBI ranges from 6 to 77 percent (e.g., Hibbard et al., 2004; Kreutzer, Seel, & Gourley, 2001; Rapoport, McCullagh, Streiner, & Feinstein, 2003) with this variability reflecting the previously noted methodological differences between research groups. The most prevalent anxiety disorders appear to be posttraumatic stress disorder (PTSD), obsessive-compulsive disorder (OCD), generalized anxiety disorder (GAD), and panic disorder with rates varying between 3 and 28 percent (Ashman et al., 2004; Gould et al., 2011; Hoofien et al., 2001). Adjustment disorders, psychotic disorders, eating disorders, and somatoform disorders occur at equivalent rates to the general population and individuals do not appear to be at increased risk following TBI (Gould et al., 2011; Rogers & Read, 2007).

Time is a critical factor when considering mental illness and recovery patterns following TBI. Of concern to clinical service provision is an apparent increase, not decrease, in the development of mental illness over time. Research suggests that different psychiatric disorders have a variable temporal pattern of onset following TBI, and that preinjury history plays a significant role in the timing of disorder onset (Gould et al., 2011; Rogers & Read, 2007). Additionally the rate of resolution may depend on the methodology used. The timing of onset may be dependent on preinjury history where recent prospective research found that early onset (defined as occurring within the first 6 months) was more common than late onset (defined as onset from 6 to 12 months), and that the course of psychiatric disorder post-TBI differed depending on preinjury status. If individuals had a positive history of psychiatric disorder, there was a greater likelihood of the development of a mental illness within the first 6 months post TBI. However, individuals without a history of psychiatric disorder were more likely to develop novel disorder later in the first year. Whelan-Goodinson, Ponsford, Johnston, and Grant (2009) also reported that more than two-thirds of post-TBI depression and anxiety were of new onset, and showed poor resolution rates up to 5 years postinjury.

Vulnerability appears to be highest during the first year postinjury with 60–65 percent of individuals having a psychiatric disorder according to structured clinical interview techniques at one year post-TBI. The most common psychiatric disorders at one year after TBI are consistently reported to be anxiety and mood disorders. In the first year post-TBI, 42–53 percent meet criteria for depression depending on the technique used. In a well-designed prospective study, Gould et al. (2011) found that 44 percent of moderate to severe TBI survivors reported an anxiety disorder, making it the most common psychiatric disorder at one year postinjury. Additionally, comorbid psychiatric disorders occurred in 37 percent of this sample at one-year follow-up.

Individuals appear to be at long-term risk for the development, maintenance, and recurrence of psychiatric disorders, particularly depression and anxiety. Some studies report a prolonged onset and persisting elevated risk of major depression for years or decades following TBI (Anstey et al., 2004). Rates may increase the longer the time postinjury (Koponen et al., 2002). However, some research reports a decrease or plateau effect for depression and anxiety disorders up to 6 years postinjury (Ashman et al., 2004). In a very long-term follow-up at 30 years postinjury, Koponen et al. (2002) found that 40 percent of their sample reported a current psychiatric disorder, with the most common being major depression (26.7%), as well as alcohol abuse or dependence (11.7%), panic disorder (8.3%), specific phobia (8.3%), and psychotic disorders (6.7%).

Substance use is an important factor to consider in relation to TBI, and is consistently identified as a risk factor. Preinjury rates of overall substance use tend to be equivalent to community samples (Gould et al., 2011; Ponsford, Whelan-Goodinson, & Bahar-Fuchs, 2007). Variability in reported rates is often related to whether or not diagnosis included alcohol abuse only, or also included alcohol dependence, drug abuse, and drug dependence. When specific disorders are reported, preinjury rates of alcohol dependence, but not alcohol abuse, are elevated for TBI survivors (Gould et al., 2011). Substance abuse is a short-term risk factor after TBI, which appears to be mediated by preinjury history. Those with a preinjury history tend to show decreased alcohol abuse in the first year postinjury, with an increase in subsequent years. Conversely, those without a preinjury history of alcohol abuse tend to show increased levels of alcohol abuse in the first year postinjury, with a decrease in subsequent years. Prevalence of substance abuse post-TBI is most likely a consequence of enduring premorbid abuse patterns and coping strategies (Jorge et al., 2005; Rogers & Read, 2007).

In conclusion, methodological concerns with previous research mean that our understanding of the natural history of mental illness following TBI is still relatively limited. TBI survivors are at increased risk for the development of psychiatric disorders postinjury, with depression and anxiety disorders being the most common. Recent longitudinal research has highlighted the significant role of preinjury psychiatric history on disorder occurrence and disorder onset (Bombardier et al., 2003; Gould et al., 2011). Individuals appear to be most vulnerable in the first year postinjury; hence, there is a critical need for integrated systems of detection along with preventative and early interventions following TBI (Ashman et al., 2004; Bombardier et al., 2010). These may include routine screening for preinjury psychiatric history, high-incidence psychiatric disorders, and current levels of psychological distress. This would enable a focus on those individuals who need more intensive outpatient monitoring, inpatient rehabilitation, and psychiatric support, and more active discharge monitoring and referral to community supports where they are available. There is also a need for longer-term professional assistance for TBI survivors and their families to support quality of life and improve psychiatric outcomes (Hoofien et al., 2001). Additionally, the factors that promote or hinder outcomes need to be identified. These would include but not be limited to social supports, brain injury characteristics, patterns of psychological service utilization, premorbid personality, and postinjury psychological reactions to disability and trauma that are implicated in the generation and maintenance of post-TBI psychiatric disorder (Rogers & Read, 2007).

Understanding Mental Well-being

Our understanding of the term mental well-being is rapidly developing in terms of its theoretical conceptualization, measurement, and real-world applications. In general terms, it has been defined as ". . . the degree to which one feels positive and enthusiastic about life. It includes the capacity to manage one's feelings and related behaviors, including the realistic assessment of one's limitations, development of autonomy, and ability to cope effectively with stress . . ." (Manderscheid et al., 2010, p. 1). For the purpose of this review, mental well-being is conceptualized according to Keyes's three elements of well-being: emotional well-being, psychological well-being, and social well-being (Keyes, 2005; Westerhof & Keyes, 2010) (see Table 8.2). Keyes' three-element model of well-being has been empirically validated in the literature (Gallagher, Lopez, & Preacher, 2009; Lamers, Westerhof, Bohlmeijer, ten Klooster, & Keyes, 2011). These three elements will now be defined.

The first element of emotional well-being is defined as "a cluster of symptoms reflecting the presence or absence of positive feelings about life" (Keyes, 2002, p. 208). In related literature the term is used relatively synonymously with subjective well-being (Diener, Suh, Lucas, & Smith, 1999); positive emotions (Seligman, 2011), and the hedonic tradition of well-being (Kahneman, Diener, & Schwartz, 1999; Ryan & Deci, 2001). Symptoms of emotional well-being are derived from self-report measures

Table 8.2 Keyes' model of mental well-being

Mental Well-Being		
Emotional Well-Being	**Psychological Well-Being**	**Social Well-Being**
(positive emotions; hedonic; subjective wellbeing) • Positive affect • Negative affect • Life satisfaction	(positive psychological functioning; eudaimonic) • Self-acceptance • Purpose in life • Autonomy • Positive relations with others • Environmental mastery • Personal growth	• Social coherence • Social acceptance • Social actualization • Social contribution • Social integration

that focus on the presence of positive affect, the absence of negative affect, and perceived satisfaction with life (Seligman, 2011; Westerhof & Keyes, 2010). In the literature, they are measured using scales such as the Positive and Negative Affect Schedule (PANAS) (Watson, Clark, & Tellegen, 1988) and the Satisfaction with Life Scale (Diener, Emmons, Larsen, & Griffin, 1985). Other aspects may include the sense of physical well-being, happiness, an internal health-related locus of control, and optimism (Seligman, 2008).

The second element of psychological well-being is defined as the presence or absence of positive functioning in life. As Keyes (2002) states,

> . . . individuals are functioning well when they like most parts of themselves, have warm and trusting relationships, see themselves developing into better people, have a direction in life, are able to shape their environments to satisfy their needs, and have a degree of self-determination (p. 208).

Synonymous terms in related literature include positive psychological functioning (Manderscheid et al., 2010), engagement (Duckworth et al., 2005; Seligman, 2011), and the eudaeimonic tradition of well-being (Ryan & Deci, 2001). In the literature, psychological well-being is most commonly measured using the Ryff Scales of Psychological Well-being (Ryff & Keyes, 1995). This theoretically derived instrument measures six components of psychological well-being: autonomy, environmental mastery, personal growth, positive relations with others, purpose in life, and self-acceptance.

The third element of Keyes's model is social well-being. Keyes (1998) argues that the optimal functioning of an individual should also include their social engagement and connection with their local community and society at large. He defines social well-being as consisting of five components: social coherence, social acceptance, social actualization, social contribution, and social integration. Theoretically derived scales of social well-being have been developed to measure these components (Keyes & Shapiro, 2004). Seligman (2011) has also highlighted the importance of an engaged life that includes social groups, communities, and society at large.

Mental Well-being following Traumatic Brain Injury

There is no research that considers mental well-being following TBI using the mental health model as described. We do not know the nature or degree to which the TBI survivor may experience changes in mental well-being as they move through their recovery. Previous research has investigated areas relevant to mental well-being following TBI, particularly aspects of the quality of life literature.

The first element of emotional well-being comprises the three components of positive affect, negative affect, and life satisfaction. Our understanding of positive affect following TBI is a significant knowledge gap. Previous research has focused almost exclusively on losses and deficits after TBI. There appears to be an implicit assumption that underlies this research neglect: that one is not cheerful, in good spirits, or full of life after a TBI. This assumption needs to be challenged, and this neglected area of research given urgent attention. In a rare study, Tomberg, Toomela, Ennok, and Tikk (2007) prospectively followed a group of moderate to severe TBI survivors, and reported that levels of optimism as measured by the Life Orientation Test (Scheier & Carver, 1985) increased from 2- to 6-year follow-up. Levels of optimism were related to positive reinterpretation and growth, and humor, but not with health-related quality of life. More positive attitudes toward disability and acceptance of disability have been associated with higher mental, physical, and overall quality of life, and lower psychiatric symptomatology following severe TBI (Snead & Davis, 2002).

By contrast, a significant body of research has investigated negative affect following TBI. TBI survivors tend to report higher negative affect, depressed mood, anxiety symptoms, and lower self-esteem than comparison groups (e.g. Curran, Ponsford, & Crowe, 2000; Findler, Cantor, Haddad, Gordon, & Ashman, 2001). Potentially useful measures of negative affect such as the Hospital Depression and Anxiety Scale (HADS) (Schonberger & Ponsford, 2010) have been validated for use with TBI.

With regards to life satisfaction, research indicates that TBI survivors tend to report lower overall levels of life satisfaction (Underhill et al., 2003). There is also evidence to suggest that gender and age are important factors, with females reporting a poorer satisfaction with life than males, and younger TBI survivors reporting decreased satisfaction with life in comparison with older TBI survivors (Siebert et al., 2002). Additionally, the experience of negative affect such as depression has a significant and long-term impact on lower overall life satisfaction following TBI (Lin et al., 2010). Continuing decreases in life satisfaction have been reported between 5 and 10 years following severe TBI (Koskinen, 1998). However, it should be noted there is variability in these findings, and that some TBI survivors report levels of life satisfaction that are the same as, or higher, than individuals without a TBI (Dijkers, 2005). Measures such as the Satisfaction with Life Scale (SWLS) (Diener, Emmons, Larsen, & Griffin, 1985) have been used following TBI and are recommended for its brevity, reliability, and validity.

For the second element of psychological well-being, research is required following TBI, which examines its six dimensions of self-acceptance, personal growth, purpose in life, environmental mastery, autonomy, and positive relations with others. There is some evidence for positive change following a traumatic event or adversity in areas such as enhanced personal strengths, improved relationships with others, openness to new possibilities, a greater appreciation of life, and spiritual development (Peterson, Park, Pole, D'Andrea, & Seligman, 2008). Character strengths such as bravery, kindness, and humor appear to mediate life satisfaction after physical illnesses such as diabetes, infectious disease, obesity, and chronic pain (Park, Peterson, & Seligman, 2006). It would be useful to extend these findings to the TBI population, and measures such as the Values in Action Inventory of Strengths (VIA-IS) (Park et al., 2006) could prove useful in this regard. Personal accounts from TBI survivors such as Hill (1999) and Durham (1997) eloquently describe the significant and ongoing challenges to self-acceptance, personal growth, and purpose in life following a TBI. In a rare qualitative study of recovery at one year following moderate to severe TBI, Chamberlain (2006) found that the narratives of TBI survivors reflected a focus on renewed ways to view the self. The four most common narrative themes related to self were regret and grief within self, invisibility of self, stranded self, and recovery in self. Recently Carroll and Coetzer (2011) reported significant negative changes in self-concept following TBI in a small sample of long term TBI survivors, which was related to higher levels of depression and grief, and poorer self-esteem. Such research needs to be supplemented by prospective longitudinal studies that include qualitative and quantitative assessment of psychological well-being during recovery. Environmental mastery and autonomy per se have not been specifically investigated post-TBI. However, related research on self-awareness, loss of independence, and occupational changes following moderate to severe TBI suggests that environmental mastery and autonomy may be significantly challenged (Dijkers, 2005; Gould et al., 2011). Finally, positive relations with others can be negatively impacted following TBI. Particular difficulty maintaining intimate or close relationships with a partner or confidant, and a loss of preinjury friendships along with an inability to make new friendships are commonly reported in the quality of life literature (e.g. Dawson, Levine, Schwartz, & Stuss, 2000).

The third element of social well-being comprises the five dimensions of social acceptance, social actualization, social contribution, social coherence, and social integration (Keyes, 1998). With the exception of social integration, these dimensions have received limited attention in the TBI literature. Low levels of social connectedness or community integration are a major consequence of TBI. Social isolation is a chronic outcome of TBI that may deteriorate over time (Hawthorne, Gruen, & Kaye, 2009). Koskinen (1998) reported that long-term changes in the amount and type of leisure activities were still occurring at 5 and 10 years post-TBI. In the late stages of TBI recovery social interaction outside the home decreased (e.g. dancing), while solitary activities at home remained at previous levels (e.g. reading), and participating in clubs and societies increased (e.g. gardening, physical exercise). The significance of social well-being is highlighted by Snead and Davis (2002) who reported that greater social community integration was associated with positive attitudes and acceptance of disability, and better quality of life. Hoofien et al. (2001) have also highlighted the relationship between poor social functioning and high levels of psychiatric symptomatology at 10–20 years following a severe TBI. The measurement of social/community integration should include both observable and objective measures such as the Community Integration Questionnaire (CIQ) (Willer, Rosenthal, Kreutzer, Gordon, & Rempel, 1993) and the Craig Handicap Assessment and Reporting Technique (CHART) (Hall, Dijkers, Whiteneck, Brooks, & Krause, 1998) along with subjective measures of perceived satisfaction and sense of belonging such as the Community Integration Measure (McColl, Cavies, Carlson, Johnston & Minnes, 2001).

In conclusion, research is required that considers mental well-being following TBI from an integrated theoretical perspective. Elements of emotional, psychological, and social well-being have been investigated to varying degrees in related literature. For emotional well-being, the negative impact of depression, anxiousness, and low life satisfaction on outcomes and recovery has been well documented. However, our understanding of positive affect following TBI is limited. Similarly, for psychological well-being, the difficulties maintaining intimate or close positive relationships with partners or friends are well known. However, limited research exists for the other five dimensions of self-acceptance, personal growth, purpose in life, environmental mastery, and autonomy. For social well-being, the loss of social and community integration following TBI is a known major consequence. However, the other elements of social well-being, including social acceptance, social actualization, social contribution, and social coherence have yet to be fully investigated. The majority of the reviewed literature is also hampered by its cross-sectional nature, limitations in the range of injury severity, and highly variable times since injury that are investigated. Prospective longitudinal studies that include qualitative and quantitative assessment of emotional, psychological, and social well-being following TBI are urgently required. The few published longitudinal studies (e.g. Lin et al., 2010; Tomberg et al., 2007; Underhill et al., 2003) provide an important first step in our advancing our understanding of how mental well-being changes with the healing process post-TBI. We know that individual differences in outcome are not solely related to demographics and injury severity (Dawson et al., 2000). We are yet to understand how recovery paths are impacted by individual beliefs and attitudes, and how these might be influence to improve long-term outcomes following TBI. The application of Keyes's three elements of mental well-being could have an important contribution to the development and integration of research in this area.

Flourishing and Languishing

The dual-factor model of mental health contends that mental well-being and mental health are related but distinct dimensions (Westerhof & Keyes, 2010). Recently Keyes (2002, 2005, 2007; Westerhof & Keyes, 2010) proposed a method for diagnosing flourishing and languishing mental well-being. Modeled on the *Diagnostic and Statistical Manual of Mental Disorders* (4th ed., text rev.) method for diagnosing a major depressive disorder, Keyes proposed a set of criteria for the determination of flourishing, languishing, and moderate mental health. Table 8.3 describes the categorical diagnosis of mental well-being.

The diagnostic criteria for flourishing requires endorsement of high levels on one of two scales of hedonic (emotional) well-being, and high levels on six of the 11 scales of positive (psychological and social) functioning. A diagnosis of languishing requires endorsement of low levels on one of two scales of hedonic (emotional) well-being, and low levels on six of the 11 scales of positive (psychological and social) functioning. Empirically validated scales such as the Mental Health Continuum—Short Form (MHC-SF) exist for the measurement of flourishing and languishing mental well-being (Lamers et al., 2010). Using these criteria, Keyes (2005) demonstrated that approximately 18 percent of community dwelling adults are flourishing, and a similar number (17%) are languishing. Importantly approximately 9 percent of individuals with a mental disorder were also flourishing. Flourishing and languishing have also been shown to be independent risk factors for cardiovascular disease (Keyes & Shapiro, 2004). Further the prevalence of chronic physical conditions is associated with increased rates of languishing (Keyes, 2005). The usefulness of the dual-factor model has been shown in an adolescent sample through the description of a previously unidentified group of students with low mental well-being and low mental illness, who are at high risk of academic and behavior problems (Antaramian et al., 2010).

Table 8.3 Keyes' 13 dimensions for the diagnosis of mental well-being (flourishing)

Dimension	Definition or Symptom Description
Positive emotions (emotional well-being)	
1. Positive affect	Regularly cheerful, interested in life, in good spirits, happy, calm and peaceful, full of life.
2. Quality of life	Mostly or highly satisfied with life overall or in domains of life.
Positive psychological functioning (psychological well-being)	
3. Self-acceptance	Holds positive attitudes toward self, acknowledges, and likes most parts of self, personality.
4. Personal growth	Seeks challenge, has insight into own potential, feels a sense of continued development.
5. Purpose in life	Finds own life has a direction and meaning.
6. Environmental mastery	Exercises ability to select, manage and mold personal environs to suit needs.
7. Autonomy	Is guided by own, socially accepted, internal standards and values.
8. Positive relations with others	Has, or can form, warm trusting personal relationships.
Positive psychological functioning (social well-being)	
9. Social acceptance	Holds positive attitudes toward, acknowledges, and is accepting of human differences.
10. Social actualization	Believes people, groups, and society have potential and can evolve or grow positively.
11. Social contribution	Sees own daily activities as useful to and valued by society and others.
12. Social coherence	Interested in society and social life and finds them meaningful and somewhat intelligible.
13. Social integration	A sense of belonging to, and comfort and support from, a community.

Note: From Keyes (2005, 2007).

The capacity of the dual-factor model of mental health to distinguish between mental well-being (flourishing, languishing) and mental illness has the potential to revolutionize how we think about recovery and outcome following a TBI. It provides an evidence-based framework to support the development of novel systems of health care that incorporate positive indicators of well-being along with traditional measures of mental illness, to more fully understand mental health outcomes following TBI.

Implications for Clinical Practice and Future Research

"Recovery is an important process that bridges illness and wellness; it deserves greater attention in the future" (Manderscheid et al., 2010, p. 4). The factors that influence mental health outcomes following a TBI are complex and multifaceted. There is an urgent need for prospective longitudinal follow-up studies that assess both mental illness and mental well-being following TBI. We are yet to fully understand the deleterious effect on recovery that psychiatric morbidity exerts following TBI (Rogers & Read, 2007). Prospective longitudinal studies that include qualitative and quantitative assessment of emotional, psychological, and social well-being following TBI are long overdue. The impact of variables such as preinjury psychiatric history, individual beliefs and attitudes, reactions to trauma and disability, social support, coping skills, and cognitive skills on recovery paths has yet to be investigated. Further, the changes produced by a TBI vary over time depending on the natural course of the injury. These clinical issues add significant complexity and challenge to the provision of effective services for individuals who have acquired a TBI. The literature clearly highlights the need for early, continuous, and comprehensive service delivery systems following TBI. The integration of current research into mental illness outcomes subsequent TBI, with developments such as Keyes's framework for mental well-being, and the concept of flourishing as defined by Keyes (2005, 2007) and Seligman (2012) has the potential to revolutionize our understanding of mental health recovery following TBI, inform the development and maintenance of appropriate health services, and most importantly to improve the mental health recovery path for survivors of TBI and their families. Future clinical research and practice would also benefit from less focus on the negative impact of TBI, and consider the possibility of the flourishing individual post-TBI and how as clinicians and researchers we can support and encourage individuals on a positive recovery path.

References

Andresen, R., Caputi, P., & Oades, L. G. (2010). Do clinical outcome measures assess consumer-defined recovery? *Psychiatry Research, 177*(3), 309–317.

Anstey, K. J., Butterworth, P., Jorm, A. F., Christensen, H., Rodgers, B., & Windsor, T. D. (2004). A population survey found an association between self-reports of traumatic brain injury and increased psychiatric symptoms. *Journal of Clinical Epidemiology, 57*(11), 1202–1209.

Antaramian, S. P., Huebner, S. E., Hills, K. J., & Valois, R. F. (2010). A dual-factor model of mental health: Toward a more comprehensive understanding of youth functioning. *American Journal of Orthopsychiatry, 80*(4), 462–472.

Ashman, T. A., Spielman, L. A., Hibbard, M. R., Silver, J. M., Chandna, T., & Gordon, W. A. (2004). Psychiatric challenges in the first 6 years after traumatic brain injury: Cross-sequential analyses of Axis I disorders. *Archives of Physical Medicine and Rehabilitation, 85*(4 Suppl. 2), 36–42.

Bombardier, C. H., Fann, J. R., Temkin, N. R., Esselman, P. C., Barber, J., & Dikmen, S. S. (2010). Rates of major depressive disorder and clinical outcomes following traumatic brain injury. *The Journal of the American Medical Association, 303*(19), 1938–1945.

Carroll, E., & Coetzer, R. (2011). Identity, grief and self-awareness after traumatic brain injury. *Neuropsychological Rehabilitation: An International Journal, 21*(3), 289–305.

Chamberlain, D. J. (2006). The experience of surviving traumatic brain injury. *Journal of Advanced Nursing, 54*(4), 407–417.

Curran, C. A., Ponsford, J. L., & Crowe, S. (2000). Coping strategies and emotional outcome following traumatic brain injury: a comparison with orthopedic patients. *Journal of Head Trauma Rehabilitation, 15*(6), 1256–1274.

Dawson, D. R., Levine, B., Schwartz, M., & Stuss, D. T. (2000). Quality of life following traumatic brain injury: a prospective study. *Brain and Cognition, 44*(1), 35–49.

Diener, E., Emmons, R. A., Larsen, R. J., & Griffin, S. (1985). The satisfaction with life scale. *Journal of Personality Assessment, 49*(1), 71–75.

Diener, E., Suh, E., Lucas, R. & Smith, H. (1999). Subjective well-being: Three decades of progress. *Psychological Bulletin, 125*(2), 276–302.

Dijkers, M. P. (2005). Quality of life of individuals with spinal cord injury: a review of conceptualization, measurement, and research findings. *Journal of Rehabilitation Research & Development, 42*(3 Suppl. 1), 87–110.

Duckworth, A. L., Steen, T. A., & Seligman, M. E. P. (2005). Positive psychology in clinical practice. *Annual Review of Clinical Psychology, 1*, 629–651.

Durham, C. (1997). *Doing up buttons.* Sydney: Penguin Australia.

Findler, M., Cantor, J., Haddad, L., Gordon, W., & Ashman, T. (2001). The reliability and validity of the SF-36 health survey questionnaire for use with individuals with traumatic brain injury. *Brain Injury, 15*(8), 715–723.

Fredrickson, B. L. (2003). The value of positive emotions: the emerging science of positive psychology is coming to understand why it's good to feel good. *American Scientist, 91*(4), 330–335.

Gallagher, M. W., Lopez, S. J., & Preacher, K. J. (2009). The hierarchical structure of well-being. *Journal of Personality, 77*(4), 1025–1050.

Gould, K. R., Ponsford, J. L., Johnston, L., & Schonberger, M. (2011). Predictive and associated factors of psychiatric disorders after traumatic brain injury: a prospective study. *Journal of Neurotrauma, 28*(7), 1155–1163.

Gurin, G., Veroff, J., & Feld, S. (1960). *Americans view their mental health.* New York: Basic Books.

Hall, K. M., Dijkers, M., Whiteneck, G., Brooks, C. A., & Krause, J. S. (1998). The Craig handicap assessment and reporting technique (CHART): Metric properties and scoring. *Top Spinal Cord Inj Rehabil, 4*(1), 16–30.

Hawthorne, G., Gruen, R. L., & Kaye, A. H. (2009). Traumatic brain injury and long-term quality of life: Findings from an Australian study. *Journal of Neurotrauma, 26*(10), 1623–1633.

Hibbard, M. R., Ashman, T. A., Spielman, L. A., Chun, D., Charatz, H. J., & Melvin, S. (2004). Relationship between depression and psychosocial functioning after traumatic brain injury. *Archives of Physical Medicine and Rehabilitation, 85* (Suppl. 2), 43–53.

Hill, H. (1999). Traumatic brain injury: a view from the inside. *Brain Injury, 13*(11), 839–844.

Hoofien, D., Gilboa, A., Vakil, E., & Donovick, P. J. (2001). Traumatic brain injury (TBI) 10–20 years later: a comprehensive outcome study of psychiatric symptomatology, cognitive abilities and psychosocial functioning. *Brain Injury, 15*(3), 189–209.

Jahoda, M. (1958). *Current concepts of positive mental health.* New York: Basic Books.

Jorge, R. E., Starkstein, S. E., Arndt, S., Moser, D., Crespo-Facorro, B., & Robinson, R. G. (2005). Alcohol misuse and mood disorders following traumatic brain injury. *Archives of General Psychiatry, 62*(7), 742–749.

Kahneman, D., Diener, E., & Schwarz, N. (1999). *Well-being: The foundations of hedonic psychology.* New York: Russel Sage Foundation.

Keyes, C. L. (1998). Social well being. *Social Psychology Quarterly, 61*(2), 121–140.

Keyes, C. L. (2002). The mental health continuum: From languishing to flourishing in life. *Journal of Health and Social Behaviour, 43*(2), 207–222.

Keyes, C. L. (2005). Mental illness and/or mental health? Investigating axioms of the complete state model of health. *Journal of Consulting and Clinical Psychology, 73*(3), 539–548.

Keyes, C. L. (2007). Promoting and protecting mental health as flourishing: a complementary strategy for improving national mental health. *American Psychologist, 62*(2), 95–108.

Keyes, C. L., & Shapiro, A. (2004). Social well-being in the United States: a descriptive epidemiology. In O. G. Brim, C. D. Ryff, & R. C. Kessler (Eds.), *How healthy are we?: A national study of well-being at midlife* (pp. 350–372). Chicago: University of Chicago Press.

Kim, E., Lauterbach, E. C., Reeve, A., Arciniegas, D. B., Coburn, K. L., Mendez, M. F., Rummans, T. A., & Coffey, E. C. (2007). Neuropsychiatric complications of traumatic brain injury: a critical review of the literature (a report by the ANPA committee on research). *Journal of Neuropsychiatry and Clinical Neurosciences, 19*(2), 106–127.

Koponen, S., Taiminen, T., Portin, R., Himanen, L., Isoniemi, H., Heinonen, H., Hinkka, S., & Tenovuo, O. (2002). Axis I and II psychiatric disorders after traumatic brain injury: a 30-year follow-up study. *American Journal of Psychiatry, 159*(8), 1315–1321.

Koskinen, S. (1998). Quality of life 10 years after a very severe traumatic brain injury (TBI): the perspective of the injured and the closest relative. *Brain Injury, 12*(8), 631–648.

Kreutzer, J. S., Seel, R. T., & Gourley, E. (2001). The prevalence and symptom rates of depression after traumatic brain injury: a comprehensive examination. *Brain Injury, 15*(7), 563–576.

Lamers, F., de Jonge, P., Nolen, W. A., Smit, J. H., Zitman, F. G., Beekman, A.T.F., & Penninx, B.W.J.H. (2010). Identifying depressive subtypes in a large cohort study: Results from the Netherlands Study of Depression and Anxiety (NESDA). *Journal of Clinical Psychiatry, 71*(12), 1582–1589.

Lamers, S. M., Westerhof, G. J., Bohlmeijer, E. T., ten Klooster, P.M., & Keyes, C. L. (2011). Evaluating the psychometric properties of the Mental Health Continuum-Short Form (MHC-SF). *Journal of Clinical Psychology, 67*(1), 99–110.

Lin, M. R., Chiu, W. T., Chen, Y. J., Yu, W. Y., Huang, S. J., & Tsai, M. D. (2010). Longitudinal changes in the health-related quality of life during the first year after traumatic brain injury. *Archives of Physical Medicine and Rehabilitation, 91*(3), 474–480.

Manderscheid, R. W., Ryff, C. D., Freeman, E. J., McKnight-Eily, L. R., Dhingra, S., & Strine, T. W. (2010). Evolving definitions of mental illness and wellness. *Preventing Chronic Disease, 7*(1), A19.

McColl, M. A., Davies, D., Carlson, P., Johnston, J., & Minnes, P. (2001). The community integration measure: Development and preliminary validation. *Archives of Physical Medicine and Rehabilitation, 82*(4), 429–434.

Park, N., Peterson, C., Seligman, M. E. P. (2006). Character strengths in fifty-four nations and the fifty US states. *Journal of Positive Psychology, 1*(3), 118–129.

Peterson, C., Park, N., Pole, N., D'Andrea, W., & Seligman, M. E. (2008). Strengths of character and posttraumatic growth. *Journal of Traumatic Stress, 21*(2), 214–217.

Ponsford, J., Whelan-Goodinson, R., & Bahar-Fuchs, A. (2007). Alcohol and drug use following traumatic brain injury: a prospective study. *Brain Injury, 21* (13–14), 1385–1392.

Rapoport, M. J., McCullagh, S., Streiner, D., & Feinstein, A. (2003). The clinical significance of major depression following mild traumatic brain injury. *Psychosomatics, 44*(1), 31–37.

Rogers, J. M., & Read, C. A. (2007). Psychiatric comorbidity following traumatic brain injury. *Brain Injury, 21*(13–14), 1321–1333.

Ryan, R. M., & Deci, E. L. (2001). On happiness and human potentials: a review of research on hedonic and eudaimonic well-being. *Annual Review of Psychology, 52*(1), 141–166.

Ryff, C. D., & Keyes, C. L. (1995). The structure of psychological well-being revisited. *Journal of Personality and Social Psychology, 69*(4), 719–727.

Scheier, M. F., & Carver, C. S. (1985). Optimism, coping, and health: Assessment and implications of generalized outcome expectancies. *Health Psychology, 4*(3), 219–247.

Schonberger, M., & Ponsford, J. (2010). The factor structure of the Hospital Anxiety and Depression Scale in individuals with traumatic brain injury. *Psychiatry Research, 179*(3), 342–349.

Seligman, M. E. (2008). Positive health. *Applied Psychology, 57*(Suppl. 1), 3–18.

Seligman, M. E. (2011). Building resilience. *Harvard Business Review, 89*(4), 100–106.

Seligman, M.E. (2012). *Flourish: a visionary new understanding of happiness and well-being*. New York: Free Press.

Siebert, P. S., Reedy, D. P., Hash, J., Webb, A., Stridh-Igo, P., Basom, J., & Zimmerman, C. G. (2002). Brain injury: Quality of life's greatest challenge. *Brain Injury, 16*(10), 837–848.

Snead, S. L., & Davis, J. R. (2002). Attitudes of individuals with acquired brain injury towards disability. *Brain Injury, 16*(11), 947–953.

Tomberg, T., Toomela, A., Ennok, M., & Tikk, A. (2007). Changes in coping strategies, social support, optimism and health-related quality of life following traumatic brain injury: a longitudinal study. *Brain Injury, 21*(5), 479–488.

Underhill, A. T., Lobello, S. G., Stroud, T. P., Terry, K. S., Devivo, M. J., & Fine, P. R. (2003). Depression and life satisfaction in patients with traumatic brain injury: a longitudinal study. *Brain Injury, 17*(11), 973–982.

Watson, D., Clark, L. A., & Tellegen, A. (1988). Development and validation of brief measures of positive and negative affect: the PANAS scales. *Journal of Personality and Social Psychology, 54*(6), 1063–1070.

Westerhof, G. J., & Keyes, C. L. (2010). Mental illness and mental health: the two continua model across the lifespan. *Journal of Adult Development, 17*(2), 110–119.

Whelan-Goodinson, R., Ponsford, J., Johnston, L., & Grant, F. (2009). Psychiatric disorders following traumatic brain injury: Their nature and frequency. *Journal of Head Trauma Rehabilitation, 24*(5), 324–332.

Willer, B., Rosenthal, M., Kreutzer, J., Gordon, W., & Rempel, R. (1993). Assessment of community integration following rehabilitation for traumatic brain injury. *Journal of Head Trauma Rehabilitation, 8*(2), 75–87.

World Health Organization (WHO). (1948). World Health Organization constitution. In *Basic Documents*. Geneva: Author.

CHAPTER 9

The Role of Psychotherapy in Rehabilitation after Traumatic Brain Injury

Rudi Coetzer

Traumatic brain injury (TBI) often results in a combination of physical problems, cognitive impairment, behavioral change, and emotional difficulties that are associated with significant disability. These disabilities usually represent an almost insurmountable barrier to a person's capacity for long-term reintegration and full participation in the community. Over the past three decades there have been substantial developments in approaches to rehabilitation, including the role of psychological therapy in facilitating more positive outcomes for individuals. This chapter provides a brief overview of the role of psychotherapy following TBI in North Wales, United Kingdom, and individual psychotherapy techniques that can be adapted for this population's unique needs to progress rehabilitation and reduce disablement. Most psychotherapy interventions in a general context tend to be time-limited. However, the impairment and disability associated with TBI is life-long. With this in mind, the following sections describe the modifications that are required in psychotherapy to better support survivors of TBI over the longer term.

One of the many difficulties related to people making sense of TBI is that the resulting impairment is not always obvious or visible. Although we can readily observe changes in physical function (such as a hemiparesis or ataxia), we cannot easily see cognitive impairment or emotional and behavioral changes in a person. However, these covert difficulties impact profoundly on an individual's everyday life. When considering the role of psychotherapy in rehabilitation, there appears to be a tension between addressing the cognitive impairments and emotional or behavioral changes common to TBI. Although intuitively it makes a lot of sense to consider psychological therapy for emotional difficulties, the presence of cognitive impairment would seem to be a strong contraindication and make this more difficult. Questions are raised as to how a clinician can work psychotherapeutically with people who are unlikely to have robust memory function, and how one can work toward insight and understanding if problems of insight are a core symptom of the condition? Although there is now robust evidence for the effectiveness of cognitive rehabilitation (e.g., Cicerone et al., 2011; Cicerone, Mott, Azulay, & Friel, 2004), for many decades the role of psychotherapy in brain injury rehabilitation was thought to be unimportant, and possibly even of limited or no value. Fortunately, this view has changed.

Over the past couple of decades, the development of psychological therapy has become part of mainstream neuro-rehabilitation. This work has emanated from both clinicians and academics, often with the initial stimulus coming from clinical practice in response to real difficulties patients were facing on an everyday basis (e.g., Miller, 1993; Prigatano, 1989, 1999). Furthermore, empirical evidence is starting to emerge that psychotherapy as an adjunct to cognitive rehabilitation is effective (e.g., Hofer, Holtforth, Frischknecht, & Znoj, 2010). Increasingly psychotherapy is seen as one of the very few interventions other than medication, that clinicians can offer people with TBI who present with profound emotional and identity-related difficulties.

Models and Approaches to TBI Psychotherapy

Several psychotherapy models have been identified as being potentially useful for people with TBI. First, authors and practitioners have commented on the utility of cognitive behavior therapy (CBT) to assist some people with TBI to manage some of the emotional difficulties they experience. For example, Kahn-Bourne and Brown (2003) proposed that CBT can be useful for treating depression following TBI. However, it is important to highlight that for this population, CBT should be client-centered, and should clearly delineate the presenting problems, identify the impact on functioning as well as activating situations, consider preinjury factors, and identify the person's appraisal of the injury (Kahn-Bourne & Brown, 2003). According to Kahn-Bourne and Brown (2003), CBT should be adapted for people with TBI by using memory aids, shortening consultations, increasing the frequency of consultations, involving relatives, or friends to assist with homework assignments such as behavioral activation and making use of in-session summaries as a strategy to keep patients focused during the consultation. Finally, it is important for clinicians to be aware of the association between self-awareness and depression and accordingly, practitioners should address this as part of a CBT approach.

CBT may be particularly well suited to psychotherapeutic work with people with TBI, for several reasons. The structured nature of CBT may be helpful for people with executive control difficulties, including with general problem-solving or organizational skills (Manchester & Wood, 2001). Indeed, executive difficulties are perhaps one of the hallmark symptoms of TBI, and can be a significant barrier in achieving independence in the community. Memory difficulties may be easier to compensate for when using CBT. For example, CBT homework assignments can additionally function as memory aids. In a similar vein, the behavioral experiments and homework assignments used in CBT may have some utility in preventing or counteracting apathy or lack of initiation, which can have a seriously detrimental effect on long-term engagement within communities. One of the strengths of contemporary CBT is its strong focus on behavior. Indeed, many principles of behavior therapy, for example exposure and systematic desensitization, can be and are incorporated into CBT to increase the effectiveness of the therapy. For this reason perhaps standalone behavior therapy models are probably increasingly used within more specialist in-patient programs aimed at managing significant behavioral difficulties.

There are of course limits to the application and usefulness of CBT within this clinical population. For example, some of the potentially common beliefs or schema people experience after TBI may well be problematic to address in CBT. For example, TBI represents a catastrophic event for most people. As a consequence some of the negative thoughts they experience in response to their disability might be entirely reasonable and normal under the circumstances. Trying to modify these thoughts or schema with CBT might trivialize the person's personal experience of TBI and prove unhelpful over the longer term. As pointed out by Klonoff (2010), realism (or accurate self-awareness) is a requirement for acceptance and the application of compensatory strategies to facilitate longer-term functional independence. A more general limitation of CBT, and probably related to the aforementioned point, is that it largely fails to address the emotional experience people go through after TBI. Although CBT may assist people to reappraise their views of disability and accordingly increase participation within communities, it may not be the most effective psychotherapy for helping people to emotionally manage the changes resulting from their TBI.

Humanistic and Existential Psychotherapies

Whereas CBT aims to address dysfunctional or unhelpful thought patterns during therapy, other psychotherapy or counseling approaches are more focused on addressing emotional issues following trauma. Many of these psychotherapies at least in part intend to help people work through issues such as loss and understand existential crises. Many of these approaches are well-suited to help people with TBI work through loss and assist them with defining new meaning and seeking long-term adjustment after TBI. Existing general models of psychotherapy are sometimes modified or applied to the unique needs of people with TBI. For example, Coetzer (2006), drawing on the work of Orlinsky and Howard (1995), proposed using their generic psychotherapy model to assist people to express emotions associated with loss and change, increase awareness, and work toward making sense of their post-TBI life. Clearly, this approach to psychotherapy for people with TBI is not new or unique. Most humanistic and existential approaches would view addressing emotions related to loss to be central to the therapeutic process. Furthermore, many of these approaches have been applied to people with TBI to facilitate emotional adjustment.

There are a few caveats to be aware of in applying these models to TBI. It cannot be assumed that all people will experience emotions associated with loss after TBI, or indeed, that they will go through normal stages of grief. Many people with TBI do not go through a process of mourning. This lack of an acute sense of loss and mourning may be related to several factors. For example, some individuals have profoundly impaired self-awareness, which in itself while problematic, may also, by default for some, be protective. For others an absence of feelings of loss may in some cases be related to premorbid personality characteristics such as stoicism or being naturally more introverted. Finally, culture can significantly alter the presentation of grief as well as how individuals view their disability. Notwithstanding these points, many people do experience the changes and disability associated with TBI as a significant loss from their pre-TBI lives and accordingly do experience feelings of loss and mourning. For these individuals, humanistic and existential psychotherapies with their emphasis on empathy, ability to listen, search for meaning, and compassion can be very helpful.

Psychodynamic Approaches

There are many different schools of psychodynamic psychotherapy. The application of this approach to TBI may not be immediately obvious. However, psychodynamic psychotherapy as an approach to rehabilitation has been used in neurological populations, including TBI (Kaplan-Solms & Solms, 2000; O'Gorman, 2006; Prigatano, 1999). Prigatano (1999) highlighted the role of psychotherapy in helping people to understand the sequelae of their injuries, but in the context of preinjury relationships. Prigatano (1999) described the therapy of a woman who sustained a TBI from a single vehicle accident. During psychotherapy, she revealed a long-standing fear of her mother, but also recognized that as a consequence of her injury, she would have to live with her mother for a period of time (Prigatano, 1999). This situation highlights the need for holistic or whole-of-person psychotherapeutic approaches to treat individuals who describe preinjury as well as postinjury life challenges. Principles of psychodynamic approaches are sometimes applied as a component of holistic milieu approaches to brain injury rehabilitation (e.g., Klonoff, 2010; Prigatano, 1999). These types of programs often focus on self-awareness and emotional adjustment after TBI, making psychodynamic approaches particularly suitable to augment other aspects of the intervention.

A central aspect of psychodynamic psychotherapies that have application in TBI rehabilitation is the focus on issues pertaining to loss. Kaplan-Solms and Solms (2000) described a 26-year-old man who sustained a severe TBI in a road accident, and how after some language and memory function was reestablished, he commenced on the long journey of mourning the losses resulting from his injury with the assistance of psychodynamic psychotherapy. Beyond the deficit focus in psychotherapy, advances in the field of TBI rehabilitation have seen a focus on present-moment therapies such as mindfulness and positivist approaches.

Mindfulness Approaches

Over the past decade, a so-called third wave of CBT or behavior therapies has become increasingly popular among those who work psychotherapeutically with neurological populations, including people with TBI. Some of these approaches include mindfulness and acceptance commitment therapy (ACT). These newer developments in behavior therapy show great promise for individual psychotherapy in the TBI population (Kangas & McDonald, 2011). Although the empirical evidence-base for these therapies is not yet particularly robust, the number of clinicians who report that they use at least aspects of these therapies in their work with people with TBI appears to be increasing. For example, Aniskiewicz (2007) proposed a mindfulness approach specifically designed for the management of depression in people with neurological conditions that should aim to reduce suffering and promote active engagement in life through the pursuit of personal goals. This approach resonates with some aspects of CBT, most notably behavioral activation, a technique well-suited to minimizing the apathy or lack of motivation that hinders reengagement in communities and meaningful activities after TBI. Aniskiewicz (2007) also emphasized the need for assistance to accept life as it is after TBI and to overcome the emotional difficulties experienced in response to the loss of preinjury life.

Mindfulness meditation can help people to live life in the present, facilitating their engagement with life as it is now rather than as it was before the injury, potentially counteracting the emotional distress associated with the constant focus on disability (Aniskiewicz, 2007). Meditation can equip people with TBI to become more focused on the present moment and learn to orientate toward an increased awareness of perception and cognition. These skills help individuals to understand bodily sensations, thoughts, and feelings within the context of TBI. As a result, some people may become more focused on the present, potentially limiting fixation on the disability associated with TBI. A potentially significant limitation of mindfulness is the serious problems with information processing and sustained attention many with TBI experience. Under these circumstances, and without deliberate compensatory intervention, mindfulness may not be an ideal approach, as ability for sustained attention is probably one of the more important prerequisites for these approaches to be successful.

Adaptations to Psychotherapy

To increase the chances of being useful to people with TBI, mainstream approaches to psychotherapy need to be adapted. Careful consideration must be given to the cognitive, physical, behavioral, and emotional difficulties many people with TBI face. Practitioners can make some more generic adaptations to individual psychotherapy (Coetzer, 2006, 2010), including shorter sessions, making use of memory aids such as session summaries or audio recordings, reviewing notes at the start of sessions, limiting the number of (therapist) responses during the consultation and constantly being aware of potential problems of self-awareness that might limit the patient's capacity to develop insight. The common adaptations to the provision of psychological therapy for people with TBI can generally be classified as logistical, compensatory, or technical.

Logistical adaptations refer to the reorganization or change of the physical environment and practical schedule of how therapy is provided. Examples of these include the provision of shorter sessions to minimize the potential negative effects of fatigue or poor attention. If not carefully managed, fatigue and poor attention can result in limited recall or increased irritability during consultations. Sessions may also be spread out over time to facilitate the long-term processes of adjustment, preventing dependence, coming to terms with identity change, and developing more accurate self-awareness. A very helpful strategy is that of using a noise-free clinic or treatment environment to limit distractions during psychotherapy consultations. The importance of the waiting area in TBI rehabilitation units should not be underestimated. If these areas are noisy or without basic facilities for comfort, people with TBI may be more prone to agitation or anxiety. Waiting areas can provide an opportunity to display information booklets or pamphlets, information about local voluntary sector support organizations (e.g., Headway UK; the Expert Patient Program). With strategic design, waiting areas may even facilitate local networking and training events.

In view of the chronic nature of the disability associated with TBI, it is important to consider adaptations and changes to the actual model of service delivery. Generally time-limited interventions followed by discharge with no further follow-up do not suit the long-term trajectory of impairment and disability that occurs following TBI. Programs may have to be modified to provide longer-term support, albeit at different intensities and at different stages of the recovery process. For instance, initially people may be seen more frequently, followed by a tapering over time, and ultimately working toward self-management (Coetzer, 2008). Although working toward self-sufficiency, a safety net, or top-up treatment option should exist in the background in case people experience difficulty. In practical terms this might mean that people are not fully discharged in the first instance, and can self-refer at any point. This top-up treatment opportunity has major implications for how brain injury and mental health sectors coordinate services, and the extent to which individuals with dual diagnosis (i.e., brain injury and mental illness) are supported by the health system (Muenchberger, Kendall, & Collings, 2011).

Compensatory modifications usually tend to have the core purpose of minimizing the effect of impairments of cognition (i.e., poor memory), but also behaviors that have the potential to interfere with the effectiveness of psychological therapy. Strategies to compensate for memory problems could include recording sessions, using personally salient metaphors to aid recall, starting sessions with a summary of the previous session and ensuring integration or continuity of the themes across the psychotherapeutic process. Limiting both the number and length of verbal instructions or questions to maximize the potential for understanding and prevent distraction or memory lapses is another useful strategy. Collaborative goal-setting during therapy can help to maintain structure and limit the influence of executive problems. Strategies to reduce nonattendance are also essential, especially where people may have significant memory problems. Some of these strategies may include use of multimedia messaging service or text messaging, scheduling telephone calls, or posting letters as reminders of appointments. Under some circumstances diary notes can prove helpful, also as part of facilitating independence from external cuing to attend appointments. For some people, it can be helpful to make appointments on the same day of the week at the same time, thus facilitating the development of a routine.

Process adaptations in psychotherapy relate to technique, or how therapy is delivered. Process adaptations change the emphasis or nature of aspects of the therapeutic intervention, often including the therapeutic relationship, as well as strategies to facilitate insight or understanding, and ensure implementation or generalization of insights or therapeutic gains. With impairment of awareness or insight being fairly common after TBI, it is necessary to emphasize the development of insight and ensuring application beyond the consultation room (generalization). This may mean that psychotherapy needs to be approached in a different way. Practitioners may use simplified Socratic questioning or role reversal to check for understanding at the end of sessions or when discussing results from neuropsychological testing. The development of a therapeutic relationship may require more emphasis, as it can sometimes be more difficult to engage some people with TBI. According to Prigatano (2005), where people have severely impaired self-awareness, the practitioner may have to use the therapeutic relationship to help these people make better decisions if it is not possible for them to independently achieve that process.

Other technical adaptations to psychotherapy may include providing written information about homework assignments or general information about TBI and its likely consequences (i.e., bibliotherapy). Where indicated and mutually agreed, the psychotherapist may ask a friend or relative of the person with TBI to help with the implementation of homework assignments to counteract lack of initiation. It is paramount that the clinician remains constantly aware within sessions of counter transference issues that are unique to working with this population. For example, feelings of frustration, anxiety or beliefs that change is impossible are common among psychotherapists, and accordingly they should have access to appropriate supervision to discuss these dilemmas and prevent an impasse from developing in psychotherapy (see also Klonoff, 2010). For inexperienced therapists, starting off by using a more structured model of psychotherapy and behavior change, for example CBT, can be helpful. Nevertheless, it is always important to adapt the approach to the needs and clinical presentation (including cognitive deficits) of people with TBI. Table 9.1 contains an overview of the adaptations to psychological therapy discussed in this chapter.

In practice, separating these modifications would be artificial. In fact, many of these adaptations almost certainly address more than one area, often simultaneously. For example, providing a summary at the start of a session compensates for poor memory, but may also facilitate the development of the therapeutic relationship. Providing written information on TBI may be a strategy to facilitate more accurate self-awareness, but simultaneously functions as a memory aid. It should also be kept in mind that sometimes, despite our best efforts, people with TBI may not benefit from psychotherapy. Indeed, it is recognized that individual psychotherapy is not beneficial for all people with TBI (Prigatano, 1999). For some people with TBI, other forms of psychological therapy, such as group-based approaches, should be considered.

Group-based Approaches to Psychotherapy

Group-based psychotherapy approaches often augment individual psychological therapy, or can be offered instead of individual therapy. Group therapy usually forms part of a comprehensive package of TBI rehabilitation, as is the case in holistic milieu programs. There are three group-based approaches to psychotherapy that can be helpful for people with TBI and their families. The first concerns group interventions for people with TBI, and includes both psychological therapy and cognitive rehabilitation approaches. The second approach focuses on group interventions for families. Third, in many rehabilitation programs, group interventions are attended by both people with TBI and their relatives simultaneously. Family therapy should perhaps not necessarily be seen as a separate

Table 9.1 Adaptations to psychotherapy provided for people with TBI

Type of modification	Adaptation	How provided	When indicated
Logistical modification	Individual session time	Reduce amount of time per consultation	Where fatigue or poor attention are problems
		Increase amount of time per session	When people have significant problems with comprehension, or slowness of information processing
Logistical modification	Length of time of input	Prioritise long-term follow-up over short episode of care	Where main focus of psychotherapy is long-term emotional adjustment; people who present with identity change; impaired self-awareness
Logistical modification	Noise-free clinic	Design of building should ideally incorporate having clinical area separate from other areas, to limit noise	People with noticeable problems of information processing, distractibility; potential for agitation and aggression
Logistical modification	No formal discharge	People remain open to the service at the end of their rehabilitation input	For all people, to proactively manage relapse
		Self-referral at any time	To facilitate self-management and independence
Compensatory modification	Memory aids	Providing written summaries of sessions; using metaphors to aid recall; starting sessions with recap of previous session; recording sessions; encouraging note taking during sessions	For people with severe impairment of memory

(Continued)

Table 9.1 (*Continued*)

Type of modification	Adaptation	How provided	When indicated
Compensatory modification	Organization of appointments	Reminders of appointments in form of letters; text messages by mobile phone; phone calls on day; encourage use of diary; ensuring consistency in time and day of appointments are provided	In situations where nonattendance is related to memory problems
Compensatory modification	Ensuring adequate information processing	Clinician providing shorter verbal responses; providing a short break in the middle of longer sessions	When people have difficulties with information processing
Technical modification	Development of therapeutic relationship	During early stages bias focus towards person's narrative rather than assessment; in-session prioritization of listening; reframing from early psychotherapeutic interpretations (timing); actively managing therapist countertransference	When people are more difficult to engage and reducing consequent risks for nonattendance or loss to follow-up
Technical modification	Facilitating the development of self-awareness	Simplified Socratic questioning; using role-reversal for feedback of neuropsychological test results; using the therapeutic relationship to help person consider more difficult choice to be made; bibliotherapy to improve knowledge of TBI	When impaired self-awareness has the potential to disrupt progress in therapy and rehabilitation
Technical modification	Improving generalization	Using behavioural experiments or assignments initially that have a high potential for success and reinforcement; co-opting carers or relatives to ensure implementation	When people have problems with poor initiation, apathy or talking the talk, but not walking the walk

entity to TBI rehabilitation, but rather as an integral part of the process (Bowen, 2007; Yeates, 2009). Indeed, one of the main aims of rehabilitation is to equip people with TBI and their families or caregivers with the capacity to live life as independently, and interdependently, as possibly in their communities, often long after hospital-based rehabilitation has ended.

Psychotherapeutic groups can be closed (meaning new participants cannot join at any time) and time limited or open (drop in) without a clearly defined end point. Among the groups attended by people with TBI, many aim to develop self-awareness and skills. Some of these groups include both cognitive rehabilitation addressing compensatory strategies for cognitive impairment, and psychotherapy or peer support groups (Klonoff, 2010; Wilson, Gracey, Evans, & Bateman, 2009). The development of neuropsychological skills and compensatory strategies to limit the effects of cognitive impairment are crucial to the successful long-term community reengagement of people with TBI. Groups provide an ideal format for developing these skills.

In terms of family members, it is well known that caregivers and relatives of people with TBI have substantial needs for practical and psychological support. Indeed, recent research has shown that there is an association between caregivers with poor social support and reduced psychological well-being in their family members with TBI and that appropriate support can improve these outcomes (Vangel, Rapport, & Hanks, 2011). There is also some emerging evidence for the effectiveness of family therapy approaches for relatives of people with TBI (Kreutzer, Stejskal, Godwin, Powell, & Arango-Lasprilla, 2010; Kreutzer et al., 2009) and preventative benefit of supporting relatives (Backhaus, Ibarra, Klyce, Trexler, & Malec, 2010). In a qualitative study, Gan, Gargaro, Brandys, Gerber, and Boschen (2010) found that support for relatives and caregivers should be accessible, comprehensive, and long-term, and should include emotional, educational, and practical support.

Several theoretical approaches to family therapy and support for relatives and carers of people with TBI exist. For example, Bowen, Yeates, and Palmer (2010) described a comprehensive approach to family therapy, including couples, with a core focus on relationships. Other, more structured approaches include CBT for both relatives and patients (Backhaus et al., 2010) and psychoeducation, such as the brain injury family intervention consisting of five sessions of psychological support, skill building, and education (Kreutzer et al., 2010). Aniskiewicz (2007) described another structured, but perhaps more novel, approach to carer support, consisting of six themed sessions, one of which was meditation.

Conclusion
Despite the differences in psychotherapeutic approaches described in this chapter, most group programs focus on relationships and a

combination of psychoeducation and skills development. Some authors have proposed that it is not the differences between psychotherapies that account for variance in therapeutic change, but rather the similarities they share (Sprenkle & Blow, 2004). The therapeutic relationship is probably of universal importance in all psychotherapeutic endeavors.

Some therapies provide skills (e.g., CBT) to manage difficult thoughts, whereas others emphasize the process of finding meaning (e.g., existential approaches) or address emotions of loss (e.g., humanistic approaches), or strategies for living in the present (e.g., mindfulness). The unifying theme of all though is the pursuit of resolution of distress, facilitation of long-term adjustment, and the psychological skills to achieve this often elusive goal.

Careful assessment should as always guide the choice of the type of psychological therapy offered to people with TBI. Perhaps of even greater importance, for psychological therapy to have an increased potential to be useful and make a longer-term impact on individuals' lives, adaptations to practice are often necessary.

Psychotherapy focuses on the personal and psychological skills to initiate and maintain meaningful social relationships. For psychotherapy to have a desirable outcome in this area, gains in therapy should generalize to the world outside the consultation room. Developing social networks after TBI are of great importance (Rauch & Ferry, 2001). In a study conducted by Struchen et al. (2011), social peer mentors were used to help relatives of people with TBI develop skills in social activities and to promote social reintegration within the community (Struchen et al., 2011). Developing skills necessary for volunteering in the community has also been found to be potentially beneficial for people with TBI (Ouellett, Morin, & Lavoie, 2009). Interventions such as these clearly have the potential to increase community reintegration, by employing ecologically valid strategies to reconnect people with their natural support systems.

References

Aniskiewicz, A. S (2007). *Psychotherapy for neuropsychological challenges.* Lanham, MD: Jason Aronson.

Backhaus, S. L., Ibarra, S. L., Klyce, D., Trexler, L. E., & Malec, J. F. (2010). Brain injury coping skills group: a preventative intervention for patients with brain injury and their caregivers. *Archives of Physical Medicine and Rehabilitation, 91*(6), 840–848.

Bowen, C. (2007). Family therapy and neuro-rehabilitation: Forging a link. *International Journal of Therapy and Rehabilitation, 14*(8), 344–349.

Bowen, C. M., Yeates, G. N., & Palmer, S. (2010). *A relational approach to rehabilitation: Thinking about relationships after brain injury.* London: Karnak Books.

Cicerone, K. D., Langenbahn, D. M., Braden, C., Malec, J. F., Kalmar, K., Fraas, M., & Ashman, T. (2011). Evidence-based cognitive rehabilitation: Updated review of the literature from 2003 through 2008. *Archives of Physical Medicine and Rehabilitation, 92*(4), 519–530.

Cicerone, K. D., Mott, T., Azulay, J., & Friel, J. C. (2004). Community integration and satisfaction with functioning after intensive cognitive rehabilitation for traumatic brain injury. *Archives of Physical and Medical Rehabilitation, 85*(6), 943–950.

Coetzer, R. (2006). *Traumatic brain injury rehabilitation: a psychotherapeutic approach to loss and grief.* New York: Nova Science.

Coetzer, R. (2008). Holistic neuro-rehabilitation in the community: Is identity a key issue? *Neuropsychological Rehabilitation, 18*(5–6), 766–783.

Coetzer, R. (2010). *Anxiety and mood disorders following traumatic brain injury: Clinical assessment and psychotherapy.* London: Karnac Books.

Gan, C., Gargaro, J., Brandys, C., Gerber, G., & Boschen, K. (2010). Family caregivers' support needs after brain injury: a synthesis of perspectives from caregivers, programs, and researchers. *NeuroRehabilitation, 27*(1), 5–18.

Hofer, H., Holtforth, M. G., Frischknecht, E., & Znoj, H. J. (2010). Fostering adjustment to acquired brain injury by psychotherapeutic interventions: a preliminary study. *Applied Neuropsychology, 17*(1), 18–26.

Kahn-Bourne, N., & Brown, R. G. (2003). Cognitive behavior therapy for the treatment of depression in individuals with brain injury. *Neuropsychological Rehabilitation, 13*(1–2), 89–107.

Kangas, M., & McDonald, S. (2011) Is it time to act? The potential of acceptance and commitment therapy for psychological problems following acquired brain injury. *Neuropsychological Rehabilitation, 21*(2), 250–276.

Kaplan-Solms, K., & Solms, M. (2000). *Clinical studies in neuro-psychoanalysis. Introduction to a depth neuropsychology.* London: Karnac Books.

Klonoff, P. S. (2010). *Psychotherapy after brain injury. Principles and techniques.* New York: The Guilford Press.

Kreutzer, J. S., Stejskal, T. M., Godwin, E. E., Powell, V. D., & Arango-Lasprilla, J. C. (2010). A mixed methods evaluation of the brain injury family intervention. *NeuroRehabilitation, 27*(1), 19–29.

Kreutzer, J. S., Stejskal, T. M., Ketchum, J. M., Marwitz, J. H., Taylor, L. A., & Menzel, J. C. (2009). A preliminary investigation of the brain injury family intervention: Impact on family members. *Brain Injury, 23*(6), 535–547.

Manchester, D., & Wood, R. Ll. (2001). Applying cognitive therapy in neurobehavioural rehabilitation. In R. Ll. Wood and T. M. McMillan (Eds.), *Neurobehavioural disability and social handicap following traumatic brain injury* (pp. 157–174). Hove, UK: Psychology Press.

McColl, M. A., Davies, D., Carlson, P., Johnston, J., & Minnes, P. (2001). The community integration measure: Development and preliminary validation. *Archives of Physical Medicine and Rehabilitation, 82*(4), 429–434.

Miller, L. (1993). *Psychotherapy of the brain-injured patient: Reclaiming the shattered self.* New York: W. M. Norton.

Muenchberger, H., Kendall, E., & Collings, C. (2011). Beyond crisis care in brain injury rehabilitation in Australia: a conversation worth having. *Journal of Primary Care & Community Health, 2*(1), 60–64.

O'Gorman, M. (2006). Two accidents—one survivor: Neurological and narcissistic damage following traumatic brain injury. *Psychodynamic Practice, 12*(2), 133–148.

Orlinsky, D. E., & Howard, K. I. (1995). Unity and diversity among psychotherapies: a comparative perspective. In B. Bongar & L. E. Beutler (Eds.),

Comprehensive textbook of psychotherapy. Theory and practice (pp. 3–23). New York: Oxford University Press.

Ouellett, M. C., Morin, C. M., & Lavoie, A. (2009). Volunteer work and psychological health following traumatic brain injury. *Journal of Head Trauma Rehabilitation, 24*(24), 262–271.

Prigatano, G. P. (1989). Work, love and play after brain injury. *Bulletin of the Menninger Clinic, 53*(5), 414–431.

Prigatano, G. P. (1999). *Principles of neuropsychological rehabilitation.* New York: Oxford University Press.

Prigatano, G. P. (2005). Disturbances of self-awareness and rehabilitation of patients with traumatic brain injury: a 20-year perspective. *Journal of Head Trauma Rehabilitation, 20*(1), 19–29.

Rauch, R. J., & Ferry, S. M. (2001). Social networks as support interventions following traumatic brain injury. *NeuroRehabilitation, 16*(1), 11–16.

Sprenkle, D. H., & Blow, A. J. (2004). Common factors and our sacred models. *Journal of Marital and Family Therapy, 30*(2), 113–129.

Struchen, M. A., Davis, L. C., Bogaards, J. A., Hudler-Hull, T., Clark, A. N., Mazzei, D. M., & Caroselli, J. S. (2011). Making connections after brain injury: Development and evaluation of a social peer-mentoring program for persons with traumatic brain injury. *Journal of Head Trauma Rehabilitation, 26*(1), 4–19.

Vangel, S. J. Jr., Rapport, L. J., & Hanks, R. A. (2011). Effects of family and caregiver psychosocial functioning on outcomes in persons with traumatic brain injury. *Journal of Head Trauma Rehabilitation, 26*(1), 20–29.

Wilson, B. A., Gracey, F., Evans, J. J., & Bateman, A. (2009). *Neuropsychological rehabilitation: Theory, models, therapy and outcome.* Cambridge: Cambridge University Press.

Yeates, G. N. (2009). Working with families in neuropsychological rehabilitation. In B. A. Wilson, F. Gracey, J. J. Evans, & A. Bateman (Eds.) *Neuropsychological rehabilitation. Theory, models, therapy and outcome.* Cambridge: Cambridge University Press.

CHAPTER 10

Optimal Rehabilitation for Women Who Receive Traumatic Brain Injury following Intimate Partner Violence

Martha E. Banks

> Women with disabilities are at higher risk for physical abuse and psychological abuse than women without disabilities. In some cases it is not clear which came first: the abuse or the disability. There is a cycle of abuse and disability in which it is possible for abuse to result in disability . . . and for a disability to be exacerbated by abuse
>
> (Banks, 2010, p. 439)

Women who find themselves in violent intimate relationships can receive serious traumatic brain injury (TBI) and subsequent disability as a direct result of physical abuse by their partner. Jackson, Philip, Nuttall, and Diller (2004) found that 92 percent of women victims of intimate partner violence (IPV) had been hit in the head or face causing traumatic brain injury. Whether a woman had a brain injury prior to an incident of intimate partner violence or received the brain injury as a result of a specific episode of abuse, she needs relevant support at many levels to gain control over her life and experience a sense of safety. Most victims either receive no health care at all or are discharged after being medically stabilized and receive no rehabilitation thereafter. The focus of this chapter relates to ideal or optimal rehabilitation as a response to the symptoms and problems faced by these women.

General Models of Disability

Our understanding of an optimal rehabilitation approach for women who have suffered IPV can be facilitated by a general description of the models of disability that influence current perceptions and service approaches. Each approach to disability informs the interpretation of legislative and health treatment around the world (Gharaibeh, 2009). In the traditional model (Seelman, 2004a), people with disabilities are valued or devalued based on cultural or religious belief systems. Historically, depending on the culture, people with disabilities might have been killed or protected; in some cultures, class, and other marginalization informs the treatment of people with disabilities (Gotto, 2009).

Under the medical model (Seelman, 2004a), disability was identified as a problem due to impairment within an individual. Health care was designed to use the professional as the authority designated to bring the person with disability as close as possible to a state of normality with little or no input from the individual herself. This medical or epidemiological model (Hedlund, 2009), with the focus on the individual as the cause of, and in need of treatment, led to the development of acute care rehabilitation programs that have saved and extended the lives of people with disabilities. The social model (Hedlund, 2009; Seelman, 2004b) incorporates the perspectives of people with disabilities and focuses on the removal of social barriers, emphasizing human rights, social reorganization, and informing antidiscrimination and universal design principles. The relative model, focusing on reducing the "gap between individual resources and the demand for ability in context" (Hedlund, 2009, p. 8), attempts to make abstract concepts practical, leading to compensatory outcomes such as employment and disability funding. In the cultural minority model (Hedlund, 2009), the emphasis is on reducing oppression, with removal of segregation based on ability status, and leading to the celebration of difference and cultural diversity. The integrative model (Seelman, 2004c) combines aspects of the various models, recognizing that people with disabilities have multiple roles and varying levels of agency.

The treatment that people with disabilities receive and the services they can access depend heavily on the definition of disability that underpins the decision-making process. This definition influences the eligibility criteria, the assessment processes that are applied, and the intensity of service provided. It will determine how people are viewed and the extent to which they are fully supported to achieve their goals in life. Thus, definitions of disability are more than philosophical issues to be debated—they are critical features of any social policy system that must not be applied without reflection on the implications (Hedlund, 2009, p. 17).

In designing appropriate support systems for women who have received TBI from IPV, it is critical to apply an integrative model that addresses medical concerns, while removing social barriers, emphasizing the right to health care that allows women to pursue independence from abusive situations, and addressing programs that discriminate against them because of the acquired disabilities. The educative component of the support systems must include training for both formal (e.g., health and justice system professionals) (Banks, 2008; Banks, Buki, Yee, & Gallardo, 2007; Jarrett, Yee, & Banks, 2007) and informal (e.g., family, friends) supporters (Banks, 2003, 2010).

Disability Identity

A critical factor in the achievement of optimal rehabilitation following traumatic injury is identity restoration. For victims of IPV who have sustained TBI, identity is a complex issue. First, TBI leads to a change in a woman's ability to function in one or more areas (Ackerman & Banks, 2006). In addition, TBI can be manifested as either a visible or an invisible disability (Ackerman & Banks, 2009; Banks, 2007a); in the former situation, others are likely to react to the disability before responding to other characteristics of the woman (Cacciapaglia, Beauchamp, & Howells, 2004; Rivara et al., 2007). This requires considerable adjustment in her self-perception. Second, victimization itself involves appraisal of the abusive situation. For many women, there is some uncertainty about their responsibility for the abuse, even though the behavior of the perpetrator is *never* the fault of the victim. The interaction of the two identities can interfere with a woman's ability to advocate for herself in order to pursue services that would support recovery. These identities can be further compromised if the woman has experienced or is faced with sexism, racism, homophobia, ageism, classism, and/or other forms of marginalization (Banks, 2010; Banks & Marshall, 2004).

Several researchers have examined issues involved in the development of disability identity (Feldman & Tegart, 2003; Gibson, 2009; Muenchberger, Kendall, & Neal, 2009). The process is somewhat similar to development of racial identity (Helms, 2007), with nonlinear stages involving passive awareness, realization, and acceptance (Gibson, 2009; Muenchberger et al., 2009). Development of disability identity is impacted by whether the disability is acquired or congenital, if there is more than one type of disability, if the woman is a member of another or other marginalized group(s), if there is exposure to other people with similar or dissimilar disabilities, and inter-relationships with people with robust disability identities or involvement with disability advocacy. Thus, for the woman subjected to IPV, rehabilitation involves a multistage, continual process of adjustment and growth that impacts on core identity definition.

Multilevel Intervention and Treatment

When women sustain TBI during IPV, they need a number of key supports and structures including

✳ Safe residence (temporary and permanent)

- Shelter
- Home

✳ Legal support
✳ Health care

- Immediate attention to physical injuries
- Rehabilitation

These needs are interconnected and can overlap in time. In order to ensure safety, formal and informal support systems are necessary and ought to be engaged.

Safe Residence

The first step is separation from the abuser, which can involve removal from the abusive environment to a health care facility, such as an emergency room as illustrated in Figure 10.1, or a shelter designed to accommodate victims of intimate partner violence. It is critical that shelters be as accessible as possible and prepared to meet a wide variety of needs (Dubin, 2011). Given the breadth of disabilities experienced on either a temporary or permanent basis, individual needs of victims must be considered. In order to facilitate recovery, shelter programs must be flexible enough to ensure that victims have access to legal support and appropriate health care. In some cases, women victims of IPV are incarcerated, treated as perpetrators rather than victims; and especially in that circumstance, access to legal support and appropriate health care ought to be arranged.

Planning for residence takes into account accommodation for disability as reflected in symptoms experienced by a victim. For at least the early period following TBI, personal assistance might be needed. In a hospital setting, personal care and support would be provided by health care professionals. Shelters providing services to victims with TBI need to consider the inclusion or provision of personal assistance. For women who had disabling conditions prior to the injury that require assistance, arrangements ought to be made for accommodating personal assistants (i.e., people or service animals [Dubin, 2011]).

Formal and Informal Support Networks

Victims of IPV can be further assisted by advocates who provide information on their rights and facilitate the coordination of services. Such advocates need to be aware of the special needs of women with TBI and prepared to assist with legal support under various country-specific laws such as the 1994 US Violence Against Women Act and the 1990 Americans with Disabilities Act in the United States, the 2008 Malaysian People with Disabilities Act, the 1995 Persons with Disabilities Act in India, and the

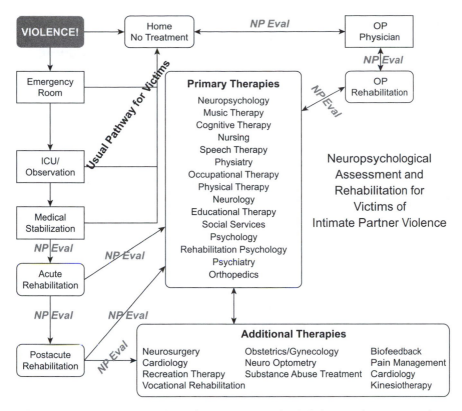

Figure 10.1 Neuropsychological assessment and rehabilitation for victims of intimate partner violence (Used with permission from ABackans DCP, Inc.)

Disability Discrimination Act of 1995 in the United Kingdom (WHO, 2011).

In many instances, the people providing personal assistance are family members (Ackerman & Banks, 2007; Banks, 2003). In these cases there is particular danger for women who receive care from the same people who have inflicted violence on them (Ackerman & Banks, 2007; Banks, 2007b). However, when family is the most appropriate source of care they are often not provided with education and skills to facilitate rehabilitation or they are included in rehabilitation to observe ways that health professionals address problems or assist the women. Thus, family members are not well prepared for the changes in function that result from TBI and find it difficult to provide the level of support required.

Neuropsychological Assessment
The first step toward rehabilitation is symptom identification and needs assessment. Given the plasticity of the brain that allows healing to occur, neuropsychological assessment is an integral part of a treatment program, not only at the point of medical stabilization, but also throughout

the rehabilitation process to determine cognitive strengths and weaknesses. The aim of neuropsychological assessment is to determine the extent of brain damage and dysfunction in areas such as memory, attention, planning, decision making, and general cognitive capacity. However, researchers have also acknowledged that neuropsychological assessment does not adequately consider cultural and demographic differences in injury and illness populations. Thus, there remains a need for the development of culturally relevant neuropsychological tests that address language (e.g., poor mastery of native tongue, second and additional languages, regional linguistic differences, ethnic definitions, or connotations of test items) (Ardila, Rodriguez-Menendez, & Rosselli, 2002; Bylsma, Ostendorf, & Hofer, 2002; Cosentino, Manly, & Mungas, 2007; Echemendia, & Julian, 2002; Siedlecki et al., 2010), educational attainment (both quality and quantity of formal and informal education) (Dick, Teng, Kempler, Davis, & Taussig, 2002; Manly, 2006, 2008; Manly, Schupf, Tang, Weiss, & Stern, 2007), ethnicity (Dick et al., 2002; Manly, 2006, 2008; Manly & Echemendia, 2007; Mindt, Byrd, Saez, & Manly, 2010), age (Dick et al., 2002; Echemendia & Julian, 2002), and gender (Ackerman & Banks, 2002, 2003, 2006, 2009). Given the specialized health needs for women victims of IPV who have sustained TBI, advocates can make certain that neuropsychological assessment is a standard component of care for anyone identified as being a victim of IPV, particularly as IPV carries substantial social stigma and TBI itself can be a hidden or invisible disability.

This chapter uses the *Ackerman-Banks Neuropsychological Rehabilitation Battery©* (*A-BNRB*) (Ackerman & Banks, 2002, 2006) as the framework for describing symptoms and suggested rehabilitation for treatment of those symptoms; the *A-BNRB* was specifically designed to quickly assess brain function, identify strengths and weaknesses, recommend treatment disciplines, and monitor progress in rehabilitation. The *A-BNRB*'s interrelated neurobehavioral domains, each composed of one or more neuropsychological function scales include alertness, memory, sensorimotor, speech, academic abilities, cognitive problem solving, and asymmetry. Additional neurobehavioral domains—organic emotions, prosody, and treatment problems—functions that are seldom included in neuropsychological test batteries, are used to determine clients' behavioral approaches to stressful tasks, predict how well clients will respond in rehabilitative programs, and determine symptoms that interfere with interpersonal relationships.

A sample of symptoms exhibited in each of the domains is listed in Table 10.1. The neuropsychological assessment will be able to specify which symptoms are present and enable the development of a treatment plan that takes advantage of intact strengths to assist in compensating for the symptoms. Given that each woman who sustains TBI arising from IPV exhibits different symptoms and that the extent and impact of those symptoms vary widely, it is important for treatment planning to be individualized. One program cannot meet the needs of every woman.

Table 10.1 Symptoms and recommended therapies

Neuropsychological functions	Sample symptoms	Treatment disciplines
Alertness	Difficulty shifting attention Unable to stay on task	Cognitive therapy Neuropsychology Rehabilitation Psychology
Emotional Processing	Difficulty recognizing and appreciating other people's emotions Difficulty expressing emotion Speaks in a monotone Family and friends describe changed personality (insensitive, minimal empathy) Difficulty relating to other people	Cognitive therapy Music therapy Neuropsychology
Memory	Problems recalling old information (own name, address, general information learned in elementary and secondary school) Inability to remember instructions Easily distracted	Cognitive therapy Neuropsychology Nursing Rehabilitation Psychology
Sensorimotor	Inability to see visual stimuli Inability to hear auditory stimuli Unable to discriminate among similar sounds Unable to recognize objects by feel Difficulty writing or drawing, because of problems handling pens or pencils Problems walking Difficulty picking up items Unable to identify and/or duplicate printed words, pictures, and three-dimensional objects Inability to identify similarities and differences among items Recognition of color, shape, and placement of objects Organizational qualities involved in drawing, writing, and arrangement of three-dimensional items	Cognitive therapy Kinesiotherapy Neuropsychology Nursing Occupational therapy Physiatry Physical therapy Rehabilitation Psychology Speech therapy

(Continued)

Table 10.1 *(Continued)*

Neuropsychological functions	Sample symptoms	Treatment disciplines
	Inability to determine where one is in space Problems with balance, walking, and posture Stumbling Misjudging distances	
Speech	Stuttering Confabulation Lisping Slurring of words Breathiness Poor voice inflection Lack of fluency	Cognitive therapy Neuropsychology Occupational therapy Rehabilitation Psychology Speech therapy
Academic Abilities	Unable to manage arithmetic skills necessary for the management of finances Problems with word recognition, pronunciation, and comprehension of printed material Difficulty with or inability to print or write	Cognitive therapy Educational therapy Neuropsychology Occupational therapy Rehabilitation psychology Social work Speech therapy
Cognitive Problem Solving	Inability to approach everyday problems, determine that something needs to be managed, identify what needs to be done, develop ways to address the problems, and create and implement solutions Inability to use abstractions or make generalizations Inability to remember and organize components of problems in order to solve them Unable to understand instructions Inaccurate analysis of problems Unable to make socially acceptable decisions Difficulty with integration of previous knowledge and new information for the purpose of recognizing and solving new problems Slow processing	Cognitive therapy Educational therapy Neuropsychology Nursing Occupational therapy Psychology Rehabilitation Psychology Social work

Neuropsychological functions	Sample symptoms	Treatment disciplines
Organic Emotions	Depression Anxiety Impulsivity	Neuropsychology Nursing Psychiatry Rehabilitation Psychology
Asymmetry	Left-right confusion Getting lost easily and repeatedly Difficulty following maps and directions from one location to another Lacking symmetry in facial features Difficulty walking Balance problems Poor coordination Difficulty with sensation on one side of the body	Neurology Neuropsychology Nursing Physiatry Occupational therapy Physical therapy Rehabilitation Psychology
Treatment Problems	Peripheral nerve damage on one or both sides of the body Unaware of deficits (laissez-faire, unconcerned attitude when making mistakes) Socially inappropriate behaviors (refusing to follow directions, getting undressed in public) Low frustration tolerance (crying out, exhibit high anxiety and avoidant behavior, unable to moderate disappointment or expressions of frustration)	Cognitive therapy Neurology Neuropsychology Nursing Occupational therapy Orthopedics Physiatry Physical therapy Rehabilitation Psychology

In considering optimal rehabilitation for women with TBI, attention must be given to incorporating *safety* into the treatment. For instance, "[Safety] can take the form of habilitation by empowering clients to receive training not previously attained; and assessment of and assistance with safety concerns" (Banks, 2008, p. 184). Women who have been so badly abused that they have sustained TBI will need treatment that enables them to work through physical, psychological, and relationship concerns arising from the abuse.

If a victim is in need of hospitalization, rehabilitation ought to begin as an inpatient. The focus of subsequent treatment will vary based on a woman's symptoms, ideally, with the aid of repeated health and neuropsychological evaluation. Treatment can be modified as recovery occurs and different strengths, weaknesses, and problems are identified. Table 10.1 outlines some of the symptoms and recommended therapies for women who have sustained traumatic brain injuries from IPV. Multi-disciplinary rehabilitation represents an optimal level of service intervention where a variety of health professionals are prepared to address the multitude of problems experienced by women with TBI. The physical injuries sustained by victims of IPV involve all parts of the body, but women are most likely to sustain traumatic assault to the brain (Petridou et al., 2002). Rehabilitation ought to involve matching compensatory approaches to the needs and capacity of individual women (Scherer & Glueckauf, 2005).

In relation to psychological processes, self-awareness training is a critical consideration that can enable women to better manage their treatment and gain insight into issues they might need to subsequently address in their living and relationship situation. Treatment also needs to consider difficulties understanding and expressing emotions, which impact interpersonal relationships and sensitivity to others. For those who have difficulty understanding emotions, treatment should include skills to identify anger and frustration in others; skills to perceive behaviors that precede abuse and the skills to remove ones's self from a life-threatening situation. The ability to express emotions in a manner that others can understand is critical when a woman is seeking support and assistance; and particularly in IPV if her emotional expression does not appear to match her reported concerns, there is less likelihood that her concerns will be taken seriously. This is particularly problematic in instances of sexual violence and relationship violence where women are often considered incompetent when reporting to authorities. In addition, recognition of her own emotions will allow a woman to deal with the psychological trauma of the partner violence and other abuse she might have sustained.

In relation to memory and recall, women who have suffered IPV should be guided through exercises to recall both recent and past events. Recent memory involves being able to remember instructions that are an integral part of the rehabilitation process. If a woman is distracted, treatment will need to focus on the removal of distraction, whether it involves changing the woman's environment or providing her with ways to refocus. Technology (Jones et al., 2006; Scherer, 2009) is often used to assist with memory rehabilitation; items such as smart phones contain alarms that can be programmed with helpful individualized reminders.

Cognitive problem solving is critical for the safety of women who find themselves in abusive situations. Support programs for women living with partner violence include safety planning, which involves life organization skills that can be lost due to TBI. Women who have access to advocates are often shown how to develop safety plans. One plan designed to assist people who are cognitively impaired is available on the internet (National Clearinghouse on Abuse in Later Life & the Wisconsin Coalition Against Domestic Violence, 2003); the plan includes documenting long- and short-term locations to live after leaving an abusive situation, finances, health and medications, other people affected by the abuse, legal plans, and a list of 10 items to pack. In order to implement such a plan, a woman must be able to recognize when it is time to leave, determine the risks associated with leaving (which can be particularly dangerous for victims of IPV [Campbell, 2004]), arrange transportation, and organize the items needed and people with whom to leave. If a safety plan has been developed, the victim must be able to remember the safety plan, understand what is needed, and carry it out quickly.

In addition to assessing cognitive processes, development of new sensory and communication skills might be necessary to improve safety for a woman who has sustained a TBI. Sensory skills development might involve decreasing visual, auditory, and tactile distortions that can be disorienting. Neuro-optometrists can assess visual problems and provide a number of everyday interventions (i.e., optical prisms) to reduce distortion and specialized hearing aids can be recommended. Speech therapy might include teaching of English or another language or developing a singing style in order to speak fluently. Interpersonal skills that are useful in rehabilitation, such as self-awareness, maintaining socially appropriate behaviors, and moderating emotional responses, are also critical to establish a woman's social network.

Another area in which rehabilitation might be needed is in arithmetic, reading, and writing capacity to facilitate vocational and educational outcomes. There is evidence that IPV leads to difficulty resuming or beginning work (Alexander, 2011). Although considered fundamental communication skills, many women have minimal mastery due to poor quality of, or inadequate access to, formal education particularly in developing countries where IPV is not uncommon although largely unreported. Not surprisingly, a positive relationship has been found between education and neuropsychological tests performance where the lower the educational level attained, the poorer the neuropsychological test outcome and vice versa.

In relation to emotional functioning, IPV causes extreme stress for women and TBI can magnify the depression, anxiety, and impulsivity women experience. Neurologically informed psychotherapy (neuropsychiatry) with recognition of the severe manifestations of these psychoemotional disorders must be an integral part of rehabilitation.

The rehabilitation of physical and psychological injury arising from IPV cannot take place in isolation from environmental change. The rehabilitative process must include movement to a safe residence, preparation for self-advocacy or appropriate legal support to regain human rights, ongoing health care, and, as needed, personal assistance. People involved in the safety of women victims should receive appropriate training in this particular area as part of the rehabilitation. Professionals must be familiar with the complex circumstances that need to be addressed for good recovery from *both* TBI and IPV.

Conclusion

Brain injury arising from IPV is a specific, but significant, problem in developed and developing nations. Women who receive TBI as a result of IPV are often invisible and silent victims who can benefit from a variety of services and different settings. This chapter has focused on some of the core aspects of the rehabilitation process as a critical part of recovering from the wounds of the war known as IPV. However, specialist services that can properly manage the deleterious dual consequences of brain injury and intimate partner violence access are seldom available and not easily accessible.

Acknowledgment

The author is grateful for more than three decades of collaboration with Rosalie J. Ackerman, PhD, who has worked tirelessly on improving assessment of traumatic brain injury and delivery of culturally relevant rehabilitation to women victims of intimate partner violence.

References

Ackerman, R. J., & Banks, M. E. (2002). Epilogue: Looking for the threads: Commonalities and differences. In F. R. Ferraro (Ed.), *Minority and cross-cultural aspects of neuropsychological assessment.* Heereweg, Lisse, The Netherlands: Swets & Zeitlinger Publishers.

Ackerman, R. J., & Banks, M. E. (2003). Assessment, treatment, and rehabilitation for interpersonal violence victims: Women sustaining head injuries. In M. E. Banks & E. Kaschak (Eds.), *Women with visible and invisible disabilities: Multiple intersections, multiple issues, multiple therapies.* New York: The Haworth Press.

Ackerman, R. J., & Banks, M. E. (2006). *Ackerman-Banks Neuropsychological Rehabilitation Battery© Professional Manual* (4th ed.). Akron, OH: ABackans Diversified Computer Processing, Inc.

Ackerman, R. J., & Banks, M. E. (2007). Caregiving. In V. Muhlbauer, & J. C. Chrisler (Eds.), *Women over 50: Psychological perspectives.* New York: Springer.

Ackerman, R. J., & Banks, M. E. (2009). Traumatic brain injury and disability as a consequence of assault: Focus on intimate partner violence assault. In C. A. Marshall, E. Kendall, M. E. Banks, & R. M. S. Gover (Eds.), *Disabilities: Insights from across fields and around the world* [Volume 1]: *the experience of disability: Definitions, causes and consequences.* Westport, CT: Praeger Press.

Alexander, P. C. (2011). Childhood maltreatment, intimate partner violence, work interference and women's employment. *Journal of Family Violence, 26*(4), 255–261.

Ardila, A., Rodríguez-Menéndez, G., & Rosselli, M. (2002). Current issues in neuropsychological assessment with Hispanic/Latinos. In F. R. Ferraro (Ed.),

Studies on neuropsychology, development, and cognition: Minority and cross-cultural aspects of neuropsychological assessment. Lisse, Netherlands: Swets & Zeitlinger Publishers.

Banks, M. E. (2003). Disability in the family: a life span perspective. *Cultural Diversity and Ethnic Minority Psychology, 9*(4), 367–384.

Banks, M. E. (2007a). Overlooked but critical: Traumatic brain injury as a consequence of interpersonal violence. *Trauma, Violence, & Abuse, 8*(3), 290–298.

Banks, M. E. (2007b). Women with disabilities, domestic violence against. In N. A. Jackson (Ed.), *Encyclopedia of domestic violence.* New York: Taylor & Francis.

Banks, M. E. (2008). Women with disabilities: Cultural competence in rehabilitation psychology. *Disability & Rehabilitation, 30*(3), 184–190.

Banks, M. E. (2010). 2009 Division 35 presidential address: Feminist psychology and women with disabilities: an emerging alliance. *Psychology of Women Quarterly, 34*(4), 431–442.

Banks, M. E., & Ackerman, R. J. (2009). Disability from interpersonal violence: Culturally relevant assessment and treatment. In J. L. Chin (Ed.), *Diversity in mind and in action.* Westport, CT: Greenwood Publishing.

Banks, M. E., Buki, L. P., Yee, B. W. K., & Gallardo, M. E. (2007). Integrative healthcare and marginalized populations. In M. A. Di Cowden (Ed.), *Whole person healthcare* [Volume 1]: *Humanizing healthcare.* Westport, CT: Greenwood Publishing.

Banks, M. E., & Marshall, C. (2004). Beyond the "triple-whammy": Social class as a factor in discrimination against persons with disabilities. In J. L. Chin (Ed.), *The psychology of prejudice and discrimination: Combating prejudice and all forms of discrimination* [Volume 4]: *Disability, religion, physique, and other traits.* Westport, CT: Praeger.

Bylsma, F. W., Ostendorf, C. A., & Hofer, P. J. (2002). Challenges in providing neuropsychological and psychological services in Guam and the Commonwealth of the Northern Mariana Islands (CNMI). In F. R. Ferraro (Ed.), *Studies on neuropsychology, development, and cognition: Minority and cross-cultural aspects of neuropsychological assessment.* Lisse, Netherlands: Swets & Zeitlinger Publishers.

Cacciapaglia, H. M., Beauchamp, K. L., & Howells, G. N. (2004). Visibility of disability: Effect on willingness to interact. *Rehabilitation Psychology, 49*(2), 180–182.

Campbell, J. C. (2004). Helping women understand their risk in situations of intimate partner violence. *Journal of Interpersonal Violence, 19*(12), 1464–1477.

Cosentino, S., Manly, J., & Mungas, D. (2007). Do reading tests measure the same construct in multiethnic and multilingual older persons? *Journal of the International Neuropsychological Society, 13*(2), 228–236.

Dick, M. B., Teng, E. L., Kempler, D., Davis, D. S., & Taussig, I. M. (2002). The cross-cultural neuropsychological test battery (CCNB): Effects of age, education, ethnicity, and cognitive status on performance. In F. R. Ferraro (Ed.), *Studies on neuropsychology, development, and cognition: Minority and cross-cultural aspects of neuropsychological assessment.* Lisse, Netherlands: Swets & Zeitlinger Publishers.

Dubin, M. (2011). *Domestic violence shelters and the ADA.* Retrieved from http://www.ncdsv.org/images/DVSheltersADA.pdf

Echemendía, R. J., & Julian, L. (2002). Neuropsychological assessment of Latino children. In F. R. Ferraro (Ed.), *Studies on neuropsychology, development, and cognition: Minority and cross-cultural aspects of neuropsychological assessment.* Lisse, Netherlands: Swets & Zeitlinger Publishers.

Feldman, S. I., & Tegart, G. (2003). Keep moving: Conceptions of illness and disability of middle-aged African-American women with arthritis. In M. E. Banks & E. Kaschak (Eds.), *Women with visible and invisible disabilities: Multiple intersections, multiple issues, multiple therapies.* New York: Haworth.

Gharaibeh, N. (2009). Disability in Arab societies. In C. A. Marshall, E. Kendall, M. E. Banks, & R. M. S. Gover (Eds.), *Disabilities: Insights from across fields and around the world* [Volume 1]: *the experience: Definitions, causes, and consequences.* Westport, CT: Praeger.

Gibson, J. (2009). Navigating societal norms: the psychological implications of living in the United States with disability. In C. A. Marshall, E. Kendall, M. E. Banks, & R. M. S. Gover (Eds.), *Disabilities: Insights from across fields and around the world* [Volume 2]: *the context: Environmental, social, and cultural considerations.* Santa Barbara, CA: Praeger/ABC-CLIO.

Gotto, G. S. (2009). Persons and nonpersons: Intellectual disability, personhood, and social capital among the Mixe of southern Mexico. In C. A. Marshall, E. Kendall, M. E. Banks, & R. M. S. Gover (Eds.), *Disabilities: Insights from across fields and around the world* [Volume 1]: *the experience: Definitions, causes, and consequences.* Westport, CT: Praeger.

Hedlund, M. (2009). Understandings of the disability concept: a complex and diverse concept. In C. A. Marshall, E. Kendall, M. E. Banks, & R. M. S. Gover (Eds.), *Disabilities: Insights from across fields and around the world* [Volume 1]: *the experience: Definitions, causes, and consequences* (pp. 5–18). Westport, CT: Praeger.

Helms, J. E. (2007). Some better practices for measuring racial and ethnic identity constructs. *Journal of Counseling Psychology, 54*(3), 235–246.

Jackson, H., Philip, E., Nuttall, R. L., & Diller, L. (2004). Battered women and traumatic brain injury. In K. A. Kendall-Tackett (Ed.), *Health consequences of abuse in the family: a clinical guide for evidence-based practice.* Washington, DC: American Psychological Association.

Jarrett, E., Yee, B. W. K., & Banks, M. E. (2007). Benefits of comprehensive health care for improving health outcomes in women. *Professional Psychology: Research & Practice, 38*(3), 305–313.

Jones, A. S., Dienemann, J., Schollenberger, J., Kub, J., O'Campo, P., Gielen, A. C., & Campbell, J. C. (2006). Long-term costs of intimate partner violence in a sample of female HMO enrollees. *Women's Health Issues, 16*(5), 252–261.

Manly, J. J. (2006). Deconstructing race and ethnicity: Implications for measurement of health outcomes. *Medical Care, 44*(11, Suppl 3), S10–S16.

Manly, J. J. (2008). Race, culture, education, and cognitive test performance among older adults. In S. Hofer & D. F. Alwin (Eds.), *Handbook of cognitive aging: Interdisciplinary perspectives.* Thousand Oaks, CA: Sage Publications.

Manly, J. J., & Echemendia, R. J. (2007). Race-specific norms: Using the model of hypertension to understand issues of race, culture, and education in neuropsychology. *Archives of Clinical Neuropsychology, 22*(3), 319–325.

Manly, J. J., Schupf, N., Tang, M-X., Weiss, C. C., & Stern, Y. (2007). Literacy and cognitive decline among ethnically diverse elders. In Y. Stern (Ed.), *Cognitive reserve: Theory and applications.* Philadelphia: Taylor & Francis.

Mindt, M. R., Byrd, D., Saez, P., & Manly, J. (2010). Increasing culturally competent neuropsychological services for ethnic minority populations: a call to action. *The Clinical Neuropsychologist, 24*(3), 429–453.

Muenchberger, H., Kendall, E., & Neal, R. (2009). Identity transition following traumatic brain injury: a dynamic process of contraction, expansion and tentative balance. *Brain Injury, 22*(12), 979–992.

National Clearinghouse on Abuse in Later Life, & The Wisconsin Coalition Against Domestic Violence. (2003). *Safety planning: How you can help*. Retrieved from http://www.wcadv.org/sites/default/files/resources/SafetyPlanCogDis Text.pdf

Petridou, E., Browne, A., Lichter, E., Dedoukou, X., Alexe, D., & Dessypris, N. (2002). What distinguishes unintentional injuries from injuries due to intimate partner violence: a study in Greek ambulatory care settings. *Injury Prevention, 8*(3), 197–201.

Rivara, F. P., Anderson, M. L., Fishman, P., Bonomi, A. E., Reid, R. J., Carrell, D., & Thompson, R. S. (2007). Healthcare utilization and costs for women with a history of intimate partner violence. *American Journal of Preventive Medicine, 32*(2), 89–96.

Scherer, M. J. (2009). Assistive technology and persons with disabilities. In I. Marini & M. A. Stebnicki (Eds.), *The professional counselor's desk reference* (pp. 735–746). New York: Springer.

Scherer, M. J., & Glueckauf, R. (2005). Assessing the benefits of assistive technologies for activities and participation. *Rehabilitation Psychology, 50*(2), 132–141.

Seelman, K. (2004a). *Trends in rehabilitation and disability: Transition from a medical model to an integrative model* (part 1). Disability World, Issue 22; January–March. Available from: http://www.disabilityworld.org/01–03_04/access/rehab trends1.shtml

Seelman, K. (2004b). *Trends in rehabilitation and disability: Transition from a medical model to an integrative model* (part 2). Disability World, Issue 22; January–March. Available from: http://www.disabilityworld.org/01–03_04/access/rehab trends2.shtml

Seelman, K. (2004c). *Trends in rehabilitation and disability: Transition from a medical model to an integrative model* (part 3). Disability World, Issue 22; January–March. Available from: http://www.disabilityworld.org/01–03_04/access/rehab trends3.shtml

Siedlecki, K. L., Manly, J. J., Brickman, A. M., Schupf, N., Tang, M-X., & Stern, Y. (2010). Do neuropsychological tests have the same meaning in Spanish speakers as they do in English speakers. *Neuropsychology, 24*(3), 402–411.

World Health Organization (WHO) (2011). *World report on disability 2011*. Retrieved from http://www.who.int/disabilities/world_report/2011/report/en/

Holistic Neuropsychological Rehabilitation after Traumatic Brain Injury: Two Case Studies

Barbara A. Wilson, Fiona Ashworth, and Jill Winegardner

This chapter describes two clients who received rehabilitation at the Oliver Zangwill Centre (OZC) in the United Kingdom. The rehabilitation program was influenced by a model proposed by Wilson (2002). Although both cases describe complex interacting consequences of traumatic brain injury (TBI), the predominant challenges in case one arose from cognitive impairments while the second involved the interaction of psychological complications and severe cognitive difficulties. Detailed formulations provided the framework for individualized interventions. In case one, the interventions focused on compensatory cognitive strategies in functional situations, whereas in case two, the primary interventions were two-pronged: focusing on strategies to manage both psychological and cognitive difficulties.

In 2002, Wilson proposed a comprehensive model of cognitive rehabilitation that synthesized a number of models used in neuropsychological rehabilitation. The starting point is the person with the cognitive impairments and his or her family. From here, assessment of preinjury coping styles, nature and severity of brain injury, current problems, and psychosocial functioning all need to be undertaken. Having identified the challenges and concerns as well as strengths, it is necessary to decide on the rehabilitation strategies. This may involve the negotiation of suitable goals that are meaningful and functionally relevant. The person with brain injury, family members, and rehabilitation staff should all be involved in the negotiating process. Although there may be times or stages in the recovery process where it is appropriate to focus on impairments, the majority of goals for those engaged in neuropsychological rehabilitation will address disabilities that impact on activities and handicaps that limit participation in society (World Health Organization, 2001).

When trying to achieve a goal, the question could be asked, are we aiming to restore lost functioning, encourage anatomical reorganization, assist people to utilize their residual strengths and skills more efficiently, find an alternative means to the goal through compensations (functional adaptation), use environmental modifications to bypass problems, or use a combination of these methods? Whichever method is selected, one should be aware of theories of learning. In Baddeley's (1993) words, "A theory of rehabilitation without a model of learning is a vehicle without an engine" (p. 235). Given contemporary ideas about the interplay among social, emotional, and cognitive functioning, one might also call upon models of therapeutic change to help understand the interpersonal conditions, such as therapeutic working alliance, or the client's experience of being understood, which optimize learning and engagement in rehabilitation. The y-shaped model of the rehabilitation process (Gracey, Evans, & Malley, 2009) suggests that the plan-do-reflect cycle, as used to support experiential learning in CBT (see Bennett-Levy et al., 2004), can be used. This y-shaped model helps to test out a person's goals, so that even if someone chooses inappropriate goals due to poor awareness, conducting an experiment to test out their perspective can help the person or family revise their perspective. Often the psychologist's or therapist's perspective is also revised.

The final question is how to evaluate success or otherwise? Consider Whyte's (1997) view that outcome should be congruent with the level of intervention. If intervening at the impairment (body structure and process) level then outcome measures should be measures of impairment and so forth. As most rehabilitation is concerned with the improvement of social participation, outcome measures should reflect changes in this domain. For example, how well does someone who forgets appointments now remember appointments?

Because of the great heterogeneity of individuals receiving rehabilitation and because of the variety of aims and methods required to achieve ultimate goals, the measurement of treatment effectiveness and final outcomes resulting from rehabilitation are difficult to evaluate (Hart, Fann, & Novack, 2008). It is now recognized that good evaluation of rehabilitation involves more than randomized control trials (Malec, 2009; Perdices & Tate, 2009).

In this chapter we hope to show that rehabilitation is a complex health care intervention. Thus any *single* theoretical account of rehabilitation based on, for example, cognitive neuropsychology, is limited in its capacity to address such complexity. Theoretical models are important in helping us to understand the nature of problems requiring cognitive rehabilitation, but a whole range of theories is needed to deliver good quality rehabilitation. The model we follow is a holistic one, recognizing that no one theory is sufficient to address the complexity and variety of problems faced by survivors of brain injury. Adherence to one theory, model, or framework will lead to poor clinical practice. We need to integrate theories of learning, emotional adjustment, awareness, compensatory behavior, and social context among others. The two case studies presented here are representative of survivors of brain injury and the problems they face. We trust that the influence of the synthesized model as described above can be recognized in the design and implementation of the assessment and treatment of these two young people. To make this clear, we state the relevant segment of the synthesized model when appropriate.

Case 1: Eliot

Starting Point: The Client and the Family

Eliot was the middle of three children in a close, supportive family from the east of England. He was an able student in school with good final examination results. His real passion was golf, and after a gap year, he planned to take up a golf scholarship at an American university.

Nature and Severity of the Brain Injury

A few months after his 19th birthday, and shortly before his departure to the United States, Eliot was involved in a serious road accident. While driving alone, he lost control of the car and crashed into a tree. At the hospital he was found to have sustained three fractures of the pelvis, arm, and jaw, and a severe brain injury. A computed tomography (CT) scan showed left-sided contusions of the brain. He was placed into an induced coma for two weeks and was in posttraumatic amnesia for approximately eight weeks. He required prolonged ventilation, a decompressive craniectomy, and then a subsequent cranioplasty. He was discharged from the inpatient rehabilitation unit to home almost four months after his accident.

Early Recovery and Problems

Having made a good physical recovery, Eliot was still determined to go to university. He completed part of a year but had to leave due to difficulty with learning and studying, as well as anxiety over the

171

challenges of trying to live on his own. He later went on a two-year course to study golf course management, which he completed but did not obtain a certificate.

Eliot then held a variety of unskilled jobs. Most recently he worked at a large retail store, working the tills in the food section for about three years, but he lost the job and has not worked since then. By the time Eliot was referred to the Oliver Zangwill Centre (OZC), he was 31 years old, unemployed, and living alone in a warden-supervised flat in a town about 20 miles from his parents. He was independent in personal care as well as in shopping, cooking, household cleaning, laundry, and use of public transportation. He passed a driving test but did not own a car. Eliot attended Headway, a day center organized by the National Brain Injuries Association. He frequently went to a volunteer center to look for a volunteer position. He also looked for jobs but was unsuccessful.

Assessment of Cognitive, Emotional, Behavioral, and Social Functioning

Eliot and his parents came for a two-day assessment to identify his rehabilitation needs in detail. Eliot had a clinical interview, cognitive testing, and a mood assessment with the psychologists, a trip into the community with a speech and language therapist, and was asked to carry out a functional task using the computer with an occupational therapist. He also participated in a client (patient) group and lunched with clients while his family was interviewed.

Cognitive Assessment

Eliot's main cognitive problems were in the areas of working memory, divided attention, verbal and nonverbal recognition memory, verbal learning, and executive functions. Our assessments identified executive difficulties as being at the heart of Eliot's problems. These showed up on cognitive testing, during the community outing, and on the functional task, as well as in informal observations when Eliot navigated his way around the center. We created an interdisciplinary formulation of Eliot's executive functioning (see Figure 11.1).

Behavioral and Social Observations

Eliot was a pleasant, friendly young man with an indentation in his forehead due to surgical repair following his injury, but no other physical signs of injury. He interacted well with staff and even volunteered to present a news item at the daily community meeting.

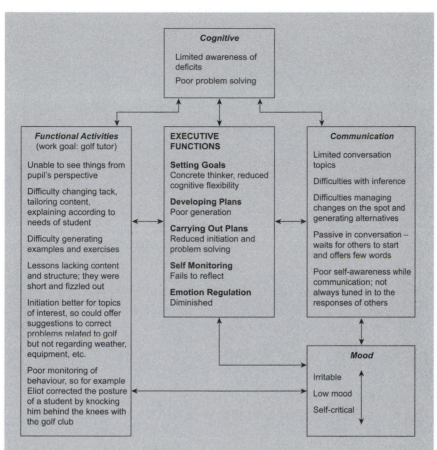

Figure 11.1   Interdisciplinary formulation of Eliot's executive difficulties

His speech was quick and sometimes unintelligible. Eliot answered questions with short responses and asked few questions. He tended to talk about a small range of topics and sometimes became stuck on a topic rather than flexibly moving to a new idea. His range of emotional expression was appropriate to the content of conversations though somewhat blunted.

Eliot showed superficial awareness of deficits. He was fully aware of the emotional consequences of his situation, expressing feelings of depression and loneliness at the lack of friends and social life, and anxiety over having no work. He could talk about brain injury–related deficits such as irritability but when pressed, acknowledged that he knew about these things because others had told him so, rather than through personal awareness and real understanding of them. He denied having memory difficulties, though he had been told otherwise. His lack of acknowledgment of his deficits appeared to be due to true inability to recognize them rather than resistance or psychological denial, as when they were pointed out, he agreed and could see the problem. He simply could not make the connections between his life problems and his brain injury–related impairments.

What Did Eliot and His Family Want and Expect from Rehabilitation?

At the time of referral to the OZC, Eliot was already 12 years postinjury and his family was desperate to find help for him. Eliot wanted a normal life with work and a family of his own. His sisters and schoolmates were getting married and starting families while he felt left out in these major life milestones. This made him sad and lonely. His parents felt that Eliot was consuming too much beer, especially when he was depressed. At these times, he became irritable and angry with his family. He had no medical problems and was not on medications.

Negotiating Goals with Eliot and His Family

The combined formulation from the assessment, the problem list generated by Eliot and his family, and negotiation between all parties involved led to the following rehabilitation goals:

Goal 1. Improve awareness and understanding of neuropsychological impairments

Goal 2. Provide strategies to compensate for neuropsychological impairments

Goal 3. Assess volunteer/work interests and abilities and implement appropriate plan

Goal 4. Address social communication difficulties across a range of settings

Goal 5. Provide psychological support to increase self-confidence and self-esteem and reduce irritability and low mood

Goal 6. Provide education and support to family.

The Rehabilitation Program

The first goal, to improve awareness, was addressed through an intensive six-week psychoeducational program in which Eliot attended center-based groups that examined issues relating to the major challenges facing those with brain injury, including understanding brain injury, attention and memory, executive functions, communication, and mood. The clients learned about each issue through multimedia presentations, exercises, quizzes, and tried out strategies for managing additional related problems.

The second goal, to use strategies, began in the group phase and continued in individual cognitive sessions with an assistant psychologist. Eliot learned and tried out various strategies to help manage his cognitive difficulties. For example, he was taught the goal management framework (GMF). Based on the work of Duncan (1986) and Robertson (1996), the GMF is a six-step problem-solving strategy: 1. Stop and think! What am I doing? Check the mental blackboard. 2. Define the main task. 3. List the steps. 4. Learn the steps. 5. Do it! 6. Am I doing what I planned? Eliot also took part in everyday behavioral experiments where he was first asked to predict, for example, how many ideas he could generate for Christmas gifts for his family and then generate ideas before reflecting on his prediction. He soon found himself generating far more ideas than he predicted just by focusing his attention on the task.

Progress toward the third goal, connecting with leisure and work interests, was guided by Eliot's occupational therapist, Rachel. One of Eliot's interests was cooking, and he chose to cook lunch for the staff. He used the GMF with Rachel's support to choose a menu, plan the required steps, and carry out the task. He selected an appropriate stir fry recipe, bought the correct ingredients in the right quantities, and set the table up. However, there was not enough food to go around and staff members either had very small portions or had to go to the cafeteria! Later, in reflecting with Rachel, Eliot identified the problem; the wok was too small to hold all the ingredients. Although he did not use the GMF to solve the problem at the time, with Rachel's support, he was later able to generate several alternative solutions that would have saved the day.

Rachel realized that Eliot needed a good deal of preplanning and structure to be successful. As he wanted to be a golf tutor, she thought about the ways his executive functioning difficulties might impact on success. Initially, Rachel and Eliot hatched a plan for Eliot to offer golf lessons to the staff and clients during lunch breaks. He was videotaped during the lessons and each student completed a feedback form. From this information, Rachel identified ways that executive difficulties impacted on Eliot's tutoring ability, as described in Figure 11.1.

Rachel developed several strategies to help Eliot overcome his executive difficulties. She taught him to use short phrases and mnemonics to structure the session and think about whether he had enough content. She helped him expand his repertoire by developing his ability to ask himself the four W's and an H (what, why, when, where, how) and to think about three key tutor behaviors: demonstrate, observe, and reflect. Rachel utilized Eliot's golf knowledge by encouraging him to use analogies he had learned in the past to explain things to students. Together they gathered a repertoire of exercises for Eliot to have at hand.

They also set up a structure for the lessons and wrote a plan for what went into each—beginning, middle, and end. At first, Rachel guided Eliot through this process and later encouraged him to fill out a pro forma. Although he was able to do this, he needed prompting for extra detail. He continued to use his GMF strategy to make decisions. Eliot and Rachel then laminated the lesson plan sheets so that Eliot could use them repeatedly.

After Eliot had practiced his new skills by giving lessons to a fellow client, Rachel set up a volunteer work placement for him with his local golf club. The placement included shadowing the golf professional and then teaching under supervision, using his own eight-week set of lesson plans. Throughout his placement, Rachel helped Eliot reflect on his performance and to use feedback to improve it. She gave clear and explicit ground rules regarding behavior, such as no drinking at the club or asking women golfers for dates.

The fourth goal, addressing social communication difficulties, focused on helping Eliot to improve his conversational skills and to increase his social participation. His speech and language therapist, Leyla, listed the ways Eliot's executive functioning difficulties hindered him socially (as seen in Figure 1). She worked with Rachel to observe Eliot during his golf lessons. She videotaped the classes to observe Eliot's communication and speech, noticing that he tended to speak too rapidly and had trouble organizing his comments in a logical sequence. She regarded Eliot's confidence with the topic of golf and his enthusiasm as a teacher as real strengths. Leyla helped Eliot improve his verbal communication skills in preparation for a professional role by reviewing the videos with him, using a golfing DVD as a model, and encouraging him to practice communication skills by chairing community meetings and presenting news items to the team.

The fifth goal, psychological support, was pursued through the provision of individual psychotherapy with a clinical psychology trainee. Eliot learned strategies to manage his irritability despite the fact that his family said his irritability vanished once he started the program. Eliot's psychotherapy then focused on maintaining his confidence and increasing his participation in enjoyable activities.

The sixth goal, education and support to the family, was tackled by inviting Eliot's family to educational days at the Centre, family groups for families of clients, and individual progress and review meetings with Eliot.

Evaluation of Rehabilitation

We determined the success of the program through the achievement of each of the goals set. Eliot achieved all of his set goals and his rehabilitation was therefore considered to be successful. We believe that we had helped him through a combination of (a) using his existing skills more efficiently and (b) finding other routes to attain his targets through the use of compensatory strategies. It is also possible that, to some extent, we were restoring lost function. Today, Eliot has moved to a cottage near his family where he lives independently; he continues to successfully volunteer teaching golf to juniors; and he and his family report his mood is good and his irritability has significantly diminished.

Case 2: Catherine

Starting Point: The Client and the Family

Catherine (*NOTE: Name has been changed to protect client's identity.) was 19 years old when she sustained a TBI as a result of a severe physical assault by someone she was acquainted with. At the time of the assault Catherine was about to begin her second year at college studying business. She came from a small Irish village and was the youngest of four children. Although Gaelic was her first language, she spoke English fluently. Her parents had divorced when she was 13.

Nature and Severity of the Brain Injury

On admission to hospital Catherine scored 8/15 on the Glasgow Coma Scale and was noted to have multiple lacerations to her face, scalp, and arms. She was intubated, ventilated, and admitted to intensive care. Her injuries included multiple organ injuries for which she was managed conservatively with blood transfusion and fluids. She also suffered multiple orthopedic injuries including a fractured pelvis. Early brain scans indicated that there were small subdural hematomas in both frontal lobes.

Early Recovery and Problems

After one week in her local hospital Catherine was transferred to a regional hospital for three months acute management, followed by a further three months in a rehabilitation unit. Since her discharge home, Catherine was seen as an outpatient by a neuropsychologist and a speech and language therapist.

Previous Assessments

A neuropsychological assessment administered five months postinjury indicated language problems including impaired verbal comprehension, repetitive speech with word finding problems, reduced speed of processing information, poor attention and working memory, problems with aspects of visual object and space perception, impairment in all aspects of memory, and executive dysfunctions including poor initiation, problem solving, concept formation, and flexibility of thinking. In addition to these cognitive findings, her neuropsychologist identified emotional concerns including anxiety, negative automatic thoughts, and depressive rumination related to the circumstances surrounding her injuries and long-term adjustment to her brain injury. Consequently, Catherine was referred to the OZC.

Assessment of Cognitive, Emotional, Behavioral, and Social Functioning

Eighteen months postinjury, Catherine was assessed at the Centre to determine her rehabilitation needs. Like Eliot, she was seen by several members of the interdisciplinary team.

Cognitive Assessment

Communication difficulties and low confidence contributed to the pattern of performance on some tests and impacted on the conclusions drawn. Although Catherine engaged well with testing, she became distressed when she found things difficult. Fatigue further impacted on her performance and cognitive demands exacerbated her fatigue. Communication difficulties meant that repetition and cueing of instructions both verbally and visually were needed to help her understand the tasks. The main problems identified were with speed of information processing, attention and concentration, memory and learning, and executive functioning. Executive functioning included difficulties with planning, organizing, decision making, and generating solutions or strategies. With regard to language and communication, Catherine was impaired on story recall, word fluency, and naming. Her reading comprehension was impaired although her word reading was normal. In summary, neuropsychological assessment revealed difficulties with praxis, attention, and memory, with the two latter areas impacting on executive functioning. Catherine's strengths were good social skills, lack of behavior problems, and high motivation to improve.

Assessment of Mood, Emotional Adjustment, and Behavior

There was a history of mental health difficulties prior to the assault, although it appeared that these had been managed at the time. Assessment showed that Catherine had very low confidence and self-esteem and was very self-critical, blaming herself for the assault (see also Chapter 10 in this book for a detailed description of intimate partner violence and brain injury).

What Did Catherine and Her Family Want and Expect from Rehabilitation?

At the initial admissions assessment, Catherine said she did not have a good understanding of her brain injury and its consequences, nor what kind of impact they had on her everyday life. She wanted to make sense of the consequences of her brain injury on her life, to study again, and to feel more confident in herself. Catherine's family wanted to help her manage the psychological impact of the assault and consequent brain injury as well as to support her to return to a more normal life and to gain a better understanding of the consequences of the brain injury.

Negotiating Goals with Catherine and Her Family

With support from the team the following goals were identified:

Goal 1. To make sense of the impact of the brain injury on Catherine's life

Goal 2. Understand her study and communication skills postbrain injury and find strategies to support these

Goal 3. Explore work/study skills through voluntary work opportunities.

Goal 4. Understand her memory problems and find ways to help her remember better

Goal 5. Feel more confident in herself and more relaxed in her mood

Goal 6. Develop her confidence and skills in cooking and using public transport.

The Rehabilitation Program

Based on Catherine's identified goals, the rehabilitation program comprised three major components. First, for Catherine to understand more about her brain injury and its consequences in terms of language, cognition, and emotion; second, to develop compensatory strategies for managing the language, cognitive and emotional consequences of her brain injury; and third, to support Catherine in applying these strategies in everyday situations to achieve her personal, practical goals. To develop Catherine's understanding of the consequences of her injury, she first attended the six-week part of the program providing psychoeducation in the context of a therapeutic milieu alongside individual psychotherapy and further detailed assessment for rehabilitation. This involved the same six-week Centre-based program as outlined in Eliot's case.

During the subsequent integration phase, which lasted for 12 weeks, Catherine attended the Centre two days a week while integrating back into her own community. This phase focused on Catherine's personal goals in more depth, developing strategies for her needs. The team met regularly to assure a shared understanding and coherent and informed planning. Given Catherine's assessment profile, rehabilitation focused on developing and testing out strategies established in the field of memory rehabilitation (Wilson, 2009), particularly external aids, rehearsal strategies, and basic internal strategies. Catherine's potential goal to return to study provided the opportunity for much of this work as did her goal to become more confident in herself and in her abilities with cooking and using public transport. Therefore, the interdisciplinary team worked across all domains and goal areas with Catherine. Not surprisingly, the speed of processing, attention, and memory difficulties experienced by Catherine affected her study skills. Given that she struggled to take in new information, external strategies included allowing more time, reducing distractions, taking in bite-sized chunks, clarifying information and repeating information.

Catherine developed good awareness of these issues and through collaboration between her speech and language therapist and clinical psychologist, a goal was set for her to use a note-taking strategy in the form of a memory notebook for studying. She was introduced to using this notebook in her sessions at the OZC alongside a specified protocol for making notes. This involved making bullet notes at specific time points in a session, with a brief prompt to summarize the session initially after each 10 minutes and then at the end of the session. The purpose was both to encourage Catherine's understanding of the information and to use repetition to support memory. Staff monitored the frequency with which Catherine requested clarification on any of her notes. We agreed that she would use the book for three weeks before we reviewed whether the quality of the notes supported taking in the information and recall. Since the implementation, feedback from staff was positive about Catherine's ability to accurately recall the content of the session. Catherine reported positively about the strategy; she felt it had helped her to be more reliable and recall important information. She had also been able to report back on the day to her father, which she had not been able to do before. Thus, by actively taking notes, Catherine was able to recall the information. Her method of note-taking allowed both sufficient information and the right information to be recorded. Finally, this boosted her confidence to the prospect of further study.

Catherine had gained an understanding of her changed memory capacity, stating, "Information in not so much as everyone else, what goes in stays in, but getting it out is really hard." She said she felt more able to manage her memory with the notebook but wished to expand its use to further areas such as remembering appointments and telephone calls. Consequently, the memory notebook strategy was developed into a more thorough memory and planning system. After detailed discussion of her needs, Catherine settled on a pink filofax with the required sections, and a protocol to remember these was introduced using rote rehearsal methods. This included a to do list, diary section, a positive log of successes section, contacts section, and a shopping list section. Her filofax was used for shopping lists, recording things she had to do, and making notes on cooking tips.

In order to address Catherine's main concern as to whether she wanted to or could complete a course at college, her course tutor helped arrange a one day attendance at her previous course. This provided Catherine with an opportunity to try out the study and cognitive strategies she had developed in the program. Catherine subsequently reflected that she thought the study day had been good. She had enjoyed being back in the college environment and had two sessions where she was given a task to do. In one session the tutor remained with her and in the second session she was left to work alone. She had felt it quite difficult to work with the tutor sitting in and felt she had probably underperformed. In contrast, when left to do the task alone, she performed better and was more relaxed. A week after this initial feedback, Catherine said she did not want to return to college in September as she was unsure of what she wanted to do. Nevertheless, the work carried out as part of her rehabilitation program suggested that with consistent implementation of strategies, Catherine had a good chance of returning to study again. She would probably be more successful if doing a course she enjoyed. We recommended that a learning support assistant should be available for Catherine, especially in the first few months or until such time that she feels she no longer needs support.

Another goal identified was to increase Catherine's confidence in herself and her abilities, and stop being critical of herself and blaming herself for the assault. A mood questionnaire endorsed her reports. Through individual psychotherapy, a shared understanding of Catherine's difficulties with self-criticism and low confidence was developed within the framework of compassion focused therapy (CFT) (Gilbert & Irons, 2005). This approach has been applied with people with acquired brain injury (Ashworth, Gracey, & Gilbert, 2011). In order to tackle self-criticism and low confidence, Catherine was introduced to compassionate mind training (CMT) (Gilbert & Irons, 2005). Given Catherine's cognitive profile, psychotherapy was adapted to meet her needs. She was supported to practice CMT strategies twice daily for two weeks initially, then audio records of the CMT strategies were recorded on to her iPhone and she set herself alert reminders twice daily to continue this practice. Alongside this, Catherine was helped to increase her confidence through a number of behavioral experiments and functional work with the occupational therapist (see below). Catherine made strong gains during psychotherapy, and reported at the end of the program that she no longer blamed herself for the assault, was less self-critical, more confident, and more compassionate to herself. Questionnaire measures repeated at the end of the program endorsed these improvements.

A graded approach was used to build skills and confidence in both cooking and using public transport. Given the difficulties with interpreting written instructions, Catherine was helped to trial recipes in which the information was presented in different ways, including pictorially, step-by-step lists with tick boxes, and short, one-line instructions. While pictures did not particularly help, Catherine felt that rewriting recipes in her own words was a useful technique. Beginning with an omelet and moving on to more complex recipes such as spaghetti bolognese, she successfully rewrote recipes and used them to prepare dishes. Her filofax was used for shopping lists, recording things she had to do, and making notes on cooking tips. Cooking tasks were also used to develop Catherine's use of mobile phone alerts. In one session, she made ice cream while practicing setting and responding to alerts. She felt that a standard alert would not give enough information to support recall of what she needed to do, and more detailed calendar alerts were preferable. As her inner-confidence developed, external support was decreased and she was encouraged to cook in her home environment, which she did successfully on one or two occasions.

Catherine spent some time during the latter half of the program living with friends, so had not been able to develop the habit of cooking regularly at home. However, we recommended that she should be supported by her local occupational therapy services to build on the skills and confidence she has acquired during this intervention, using the strategy of rewriting recipes in her own words, trialing them (crossing off steps with a highlighter as they have been completed) and adjusting them if necessary.

Catherine lacked confidence in using public transport in unfamiliar areas for fear of getting lost. She was accompanied on a trip into Cambridge (a 15-minute train ride away), during which she was shown the procedure of finding train times, buying tickets, finding the correct platform, and using landmarks to navigate to a destination at the other end. The filofax was used to support recall of this information. The following week, Catherine repeated the journey with a therapist shadowing (i.e., accompanying her and not directing). While she reported feeling apprehensive about it, Catherine carried out the journey successfully, and felt satisfied with her performance. To develop her confidence further, we recommended that she receive ongoing support from an occupational therapist to carry on making journeys in her local area.

Catherine's final challenge was to plan, shop for and prepare a farewell lunch for the rest of her fellow clients. This task served as a vehicle for bringing together various areas of work, including use of the filofax, cooking skills, recipe adaptation, using public transport, and route finding. Catherine coped extremely well with a more complex recipe, and displayed increased confidence compared with the early days of the program. She sought assistance from the therapist on fewer occasions, and independently problem-solved more than once. Catherine received good feedback from her fellow clients, and reported feeling proud of herself for this achievement.

To support Catherine in identifying possible areas of interest with regard to work/study, a work placement was arranged for her in a local clinic assisting elderly people. She spent 90 minutes twice a week shadowing staff delivering groups and administering one-to-one exercise program. Feedback from the placement was extremely positive. Catherine was said to fit in well, to be extremely personable and to interact pleasantly and appropriately with staff and clients. While Catherine now feels that she would prefer not to work with older people, she felt that the placement had given her more confidence in her ability to interact with others. It was recommended that Catherine be supported to engage in a more taxing placement, to offer opportunities to be more actively involved in work-related tasks. This could be beneficial for her to experience a range of different roles—whether paid or voluntary—to facilitate a decision about her future vocational plans.

Another element of the program involved the provision of education on understanding brain injury to Catherine's family. The family reflected that this had developed their own understanding of Catherine's brain injury as well as helping them to adjust to these consequences.

Evaluation of Rehabilitation

Like Eliot, Catherine achieved the goals set. Performance was monitored throughout and the program considered successful by Catherine and her family. We used models from memory therapy, executive rehabilitation, and psychotherapy to help Catherine use her existing skills more efficiently and compensate for her deficits. She is currently helping out a family member with their family business for a short period of time and is also keen to pursue living independently.

Conclusion

In this chapter we have described a synthesized model used to plan rehabilitation for people with acquired nonprogressive brain injury, illustrated through two case studies. The first case study described Eliot, a young man who sustained a TBI in a motor vehicle accident and was left with major cognitive difficulties. The second case was Catherine, a young woman who survived a serious assault, leaving her with significant emotional problems in addition to cognitive impairments.

Following Wilson's (2002) model, the starting point for rehabilitation is always the patient and the family, what they want and hope to achieve from rehabilitation. Their understanding about the brain injury and its consequences is crucial in the process. Eliot and his family and Catherine and her family were very involved in their rehabilitation. We aimed to understand the preinjury coping styles, mental health, social and ethnic background, and lifestyles of these two young people as well as the nature, extent, and severity of the brain damage. We assessed their cognitive, emotional, behavioral, and social functioning in order to identify their problems. Together with the clients and their families, we developed relevant and meaningful goals, which we enabled the clients achieve through a number of strategies from cognitive rehabilitation and psychotherapy. We evaluated success through measuring change in everyday behavior. We were implicitly influenced by a variety of theories and we worked closely as a multidisciplinary and interdisciplinary team.

Eliot and Catherine still have difficulties and we need to remember that rehabilitation is not synonymous with recovery. Nevertheless, they have been enabled to move forward and participate in areas of life previously denied to them because of their deficits. Our hope is that all survivors of brain injury are given similar opportunities to achieve their maximum potential.

References

Ashworth, F., Gracey, F., & Gilbert, P. (2011). Compassion focused therapy after traumatic brain injury: Theoretical foundations and a case illustration. *Brain Impairment, 12*(2), 128–139.

Baddeley, A. (1993). A theory of rehabilitation without a model of learning is a vehicle without an engine: a comment on Caramazza and Hillis. *Neuropsychological Rehabilitation, 3*(3), 235–244.

Bennett-Levy, J., Butler, G., Fennell, M., Hackmann, A., Mueller, M., & Westbrook, D. (2004). *Oxford guide to behavioral experiments in cognitive therapy*. Oxford: Oxford University Press.

Duncan, J. (1986). Disorganization of behaviour after frontal lobe damage. *Cognitive Neuropsychology, 3*(3), 271–290.

Gilbert, P., & Irons, C. (2005). Focused therapies and compassionate mind training for shame and self-attacking. In P. Gilbert (Ed.), *Compassion: Conceptualisations, research and use in psychotherapy* (pp. 263–325). Hove, East Sussex: Routledge.

Gracey, F., Evans, J. J., & Malley, D. (2009). Capturing process and outcome in complex rehabilitation interventions: a "Y" shaped model. *Neuropsychological Rehabilitation, 19*(6), 867–890.

Gracey, F., & Ownsworth, T. (2008). The self and identity in rehabilitation. *Neuropsychological Rehabilitation, 18*, 522–526.

Hart, T., Fann, J. R., & Novack, T. A. (2008). The dilemma of the control condition in experience-based cognitive and behavioral treatment research. *Neuropsychological Rehabilitation, 18*(1), 1–21.

Malec, J. F. (2009). New methodologies for intervention and outcome measurement. *Neuropsychological Rehabilitation, 19*, 785–806.

Perdices, M., & Tate, R. L. (2009). Single subject designs as a tool for evidence-based practice: Are they unrecognized and undervalued? *Neuropsychological Rehabilitation, 19*(6), 904–927.

Robertson, I. H. (1996). *Goal management training: a clinical manual.* Cambridge: PsyConsult.

Whyte, J. (1997). Distinctive methodologic challenges. In M. J. Fuhrer (Ed.), *Assessing medical rehabilitation practices: the promise of outcomes research.* Baltimore, MD: Paul H. Brookes Publishing Co.

Wilson, B. A. (2002). Towards a comprehensive model of cognitive rehabilitation. *Neuropsychological Rehabilitation, 12*(2), 97–110.

Wilson, B.A. (2009). *Memory rehabilitation: Integrating theory and practice.* New York: Guilford Press.

World Health Organization (WHO). (2001). *International classification of functioning, disability and health.* Geneva: WHO.

PART 4

PLACES, COMMUNITIES, AND CULTURES: DRAWING ON THE STRENGTH OF MANY

Heidi Muenchberger

There is, and perhaps cannot be, a single or simple model of traumatic brain injury rehabilitation delivered in Australia or internationally. Settings are diverse, practitioners are variable in their approaches, cultures are distinctly different, communities respond to particular local priorities, and research is far from complete when considering the best model components. Most importantly, individuals all differ in their own unique way.

Although it is expected that brain injury service delivery may vary across cultures and contexts, the aspirations and goals of people with brain injury, and those of others who facilitate their outcomes (i.e., health professionals, families, carers) are often similar. As poignantly stated by Alexander Chalmers, the 18th-century Scottish writer, editor, and doctor, "the grand essentials of happiness are: something to do, something to love and something to hope for." In this regard, the aspirations of people living with brain injury or any other chronic or significant illness or injury are not likely to differ from those of the general population. So, how do we build environments that can support people to reach such lofty goals? What types of systems can acknowledge the diversity that is inherent in the population at the same time as recognizing the important similarities across people and not marginalizing those who have been labeled as having a disability?

Thankfully, we have moved beyond individualistic models of recovery that focus solely on the person and their deficits. Through important movements such as the International Classification of Functioning and Disability (ICF—WHO, 2001), which reflects a broad biopsychosocial philosophy, we have come to recognize the role of personal circumstances as well as social contexts and environmental supports. In other sectors, this shift has led to a focus on the social determinants of health (e.g., Shultz & Northridge, 2004). This approach acknowledges the critical environmental factors that shape our health and well-being, such as the communities in which we live and work, the places we call home, and the impact of those with whom we live. Indeed, community is the best place from which to facilitate meaningful change for people with brain injury. Although community comes in many different shapes and can mean different things, in its broader sense, it is often an underutilized source of real-world support for people who have been damaged in some way. Strong support in the community can lead to a sense of belonging, social identity, and self-worth, factors that are essential to the process of rebuilding well-being.

This section of the book relates to the significance of place, community, and culture, and the intersection of these elements. It describes the meaning of home as a psychological concept and marker of personal identity. Housing and in-home support remain principal areas of unmet need for people living with brain injury. Indeed, those most in need of quality housing and healing environments are usually also those who are at greatest risk of limited housing choice and poor health outcomes. They often experience unstable housing situations with multiple periods of short-term tenancy, heavy reliance on last resort housing and, at worst, homelessness. Thus, a sense of belonging in place is a fundamental concept to regain after brain injury, particularly following upheaval, uncertainty, and changing capacity and resources for both the individual and families involved.

International models of community-based rehabilitation capitalize on the capacity of communities to develop local solutions that can address resource constraints. Peer networks (i.e., natural supports) located within community are a silent volunteer army constructed from those who are most likely to accompany the person on their lifelong journey. Without the support of these grassroots community networks, brain injury rehabilitation becomes a much longer and lonelier experience. Health professionals and formal services cannot fill the gaps these networks address.

Health care for people with chronic conditions is embedded within a wider social and support system (Wilson, Holt, & Greenhalgh, 2001). For many people with brain injury, the outcomes of rehabilitation depend on the activation of key triggers, usually associated with the presence or absence of critical events including the following:

* The transition from hospital to home and the associated loss of structure
* The coordination of care across services given that the rehabilitation continuum is little more than a collection of disjointed parts

* Access to individualized funding to support the receipt of timely services and equipment
* Experiences of culturally responsive (or unresponsive) services
* The provision of structured support for families versus the failure to capitalize on natural supports
* The availability of community housing options that overcome the persistent focus on short-term care arrangements rather than life course planning
* Facilitation of meaningful vocational options and opportunities.

When these events are experienced as being negative, inadequate, or inappropriate, any number of outcomes becomes possible, usually deleterious, but clearly preventable. Indeed, there is evidence that rehabilitation systems can act as agents of harm rather than healing if attention is not given to the way in which these environmental and contextual factors are addressed (Kendall & Muenchberger, 2009).

Crisis-driven care is the antithesis of rehabilitation that maximizes opportunities for growth and secures positive long-term outcomes. Innovative solutions for moving beyond the reactive approach to brain injury rehabilitation are crucial for optimizing outcomes in this area. People living with brain injury typically have many productive and quality years ahead of them. However, by only attending to immediate and short-term care needs rather than the broader environmental influences, we are at risk of limiting the capacity of individuals to fully explore their postinjury capabilities, regain their confidence, and flourish within the community despite their disability.

References

Kendall, E., & Muenchberger, H. (2009). When systems hurt rather than heal: Outcomes following psychological injury at work. In Marshall C., Kendall E., Gover, R., Banks M. (Eds.). *Volume 3: Disability: Insights from across fields and around the world* (pp. 145–154). Westport, CT: Praeger.

Schulz, A., & Northridge, M. E. (2004). Social determinants of health and environmental health promotion. *Health Education and Behavior, 31,*455–471.

WHO (2001). International classification of functioning, disability and health, from http://www.who.int/classifications/icf/en/

Wilson, T., Holt, T., & Greenhalgh, T. (2001). Complexity science: Complexity and clinical care. *British Medical Journal, 323,* 685–688.

STAND

I learned how to stand
From a man who sits
To rise above the odds—And
Speak words with no hidden rhyme.
I learned to stand and move swiftly in a dance
For I can stand when given a chance
I learned how to move change and grow
All from a man I saw blessed by the Pope.
To breathe the air of old Roman streets
Led by The Professor who could not use his feet.
To stand is in mind, wisdom—Fruitful awareness
To stand is the heart—Courage of lions
I learned to stand for myself
Body and mind
From man who sits all the time.
I learned to stand and push for more
From a man who taught Siddhartha, feet not touching the flour.
Following his lead down the coble stone streets
I learned,
There is no place I cannot go
And Stand.

Erica Anderson

"There's No Place Like Home": The Experience of Home for Young People with Acquired Brain Injury in Residential Care Environments

Hayley Danielle Quinn

It was dreadful, I was just stuck in my room all day, I had no interaction with anybody. If I wanted a nurse I had to call for one. I wasn't given any physio [therapy], well, there was a physiotherapist there but he only came in if he wanted to work all day, so that was very rarely. So I was just stuck in a room all day. I didn't even . . . I think I had . . ., my mum bought me in a small TV in the end so I could watch a bit of TV. I was just stuck in the room all day, nobody to talk to because everybody there was very old, half of them couldn't talk. So I was just stuck in the room all day and that was it . . . people did not like to come and visit . . . I didn't have any of my things about. There was nowhere to put anything you wanted. Just one room and that was it . . . It was horrible, very, very—you felt ostracized, you felt like an outcast. It was horrible.

(Quote from an interview with Freda)

For a long time, service providers have been linking the word home— whether it be home, homely, or homelike—to residential care environments for people with acquired brain injury (ABI) (Annison, 2000). This connection is often made without an in-depth understanding of what a home embodies for this population. According to Annison (2000), it is important to identify the perceptions of the individuals who live within a particular environment in order to understand what constitutes a home for that group of people. Without this subjective knowledge, it will be difficult to provide services that optimize quality of life.

In demonstrating how home can contribute to quality of life, Annison (2000) utilized Maslow's (1943) hierarchy of needs as a way of developing a multifaceted approach to creating and maintaining home environments. Maslow's three classifications of need are: (1) fundamental needs, such as the physiological needs for water, food, warmth, and shelter; (2) intermediate needs, such as the need for security, safety, love and affection, belongingness, social acceptance, and self-esteem; and (3) growth needs, including the need for creativity, self-actualization, justice, goodness, beauty, order, and unity. The home can meet fundamental needs through the provision of shelter and a place to engage in activities such as sleeping. Other elements of the home can meet intermediate needs such as belongingness, safety, privacy, and an emotionally supportive environment. Finally, individual's growth needs can be met through the tasks associated with taking responsibility for the home, managing one's behavior in the home, and manipulating one's environment to suit one's needs, and providing opportunities for self-expression. Meeting these needs is integral to a person's well-being, implying that home can be one of the most important contributors to individual development and adjustment (Annison, 2000). Annison (2000) concluded that the concept of home contained many features. Although no single feature alone enables the realization of a true home, the absence of any one of these features may transform the space into a *nonhome*.

Stedman's (2002) research similarly confirmed that the meanings ascribed to a place are important determinants of attachment, satisfaction, and behaviors. Thus, the physical place is a center where meaning is constructed (Tuan, 1977). This sense of place can be seen as an individual's or group's collection of symbolic meanings, satisfaction with, and attachment to a spatial setting (Stedman, 2002). Satisfaction is derived from the functional value of a place to meet a range of basic needs including services, sociability, and physical characteristics (Stedman, 2002). As Ridgway, Simpson, Wittman, and Wheeler (1994) stated,

> Empowerment is often found in the details of the mundane world. It comes from controlling access to personal space, from being able to alter one's environment and select one's daily routine, and from having personal space that reflects and upholds one's identity and interests (p. 413).

Home may actually become increasingly significant for people whose geographical and social worlds have decreased in size due to illness or mobility issues (Dyck, Kontos, Angus, & McKeever, 2005). Thus, when disability necessitates the provision of care services, particularly medical or adaptive equipment, within the home, routine activities and the established meanings of the home can be disrupted (Dyck et al., 2005; Ruddick, 1995; Tamm, 1999). In this situation, home also becomes a workplace for paid caregivers. The provision of care services disrupts the meaning of home and challenges not only the person's privacy, but also his or her identity (Dyck et al., 2005). This complex dynamic highlights the importance of ensuring that individuals care needs are met safely at the same time as maintaining their control over their own environment, and their sense of identity in that place.

The majority of studies focusing on the meaning of home have involved the general population and individuals without a recognized disability. So what does home mean for people with acquired brain injury (ABI) who can no longer be cared for in the home of their choice and reside in a residential environment providing full-time (24 hours/7days) support? Quality of life benefits have been found to only accrue when the holistic features of home are present, which indicates that the quest for quality may be complicated by the residential environment in which the person finds themselves. Therefore, it is necessary to ensure that service providers take into account this multifaceted character of home when providing accommodation for people with ABI (Muenchberger, Ehrlich, Kendall, & Vit, 2012). In this chapter, the lives of two individuals with ABI will be explored to understand their meaning of home following movement to a purpose-built residential facility. The selected residents applied through an independent housing referral process to reside in the new accommodation with other people who were living with multiple sclerosis and other degenerative neurological disorders.

The new residential facility was designed to offer private, self-contained apartments for younger people (i.e., less than 65 years of age) with access to full-time nursing and attendant support. This physical design of the apartments aimed to provide residents with the choice to maintain their privacy and remain within their own apartments, having all the necessary facilities for sleeping, cooking, personal hygiene, and entertainment, or to access spaces within the building to spend time with other residents and staff. The apartments were designed to provide a more home-like environment for residents and visiting family members, with separate rooms and living space unlike that found in other residential environments where only a private bedroom area is provided.

This chapter identifies the experience of home for these two residents and the way in which they interpreted the sense of place. Each resident spent several hours talking about the notion of home during the first 12 months after voluntarily moving into their new accommodation. These discussions, and where appropriate, their own words, form the material that is contained in this chapter. Throughout the chapter, the new accommodation is referred to as Mei Domus, meaning my home in Latin.

Freda

Freda (*name changed to protect the identity of the client) is a female resident who was 52 years of age and had been living at Mei Domus for 6 to 8 months. At the time of her brain aneurysm in 2002, she was married with three children aged between 17 and 23 years. Following her brain injury, her marriage soon ended and divorce ensued. At the time of her injury, Freda was responsible for maintaining home duties, she led a busy and active life, and was involved in competitive sport. Following her discharge from hospital she lived with her mother and was later transferred to a residential aged care facility where she lived for two years prior to moving to Mei Domus.

Since moving to Mei Domus, Freda receives regular weekly visits from her mother and semiregular (three times weekly) visits from her children. She has frequent telephone and e-mail contact with family and friends. The availability of and accessibility to communication technology within her apartment has allowed Freda to stay in contact with family and friends. Previously, she did not have access to a private telephone so had to make calls in the public area of the residential facility: "I didn't have a phone in my room at [previous accommodation]. I had to go out to the public area and try and get a phone there. I have a phone in my room here, it's easy." There is the option at Mei Domus for family or friends to stay overnight, and whilst this has not yet happened for Freda, she often talks about her plans for friends to come and stay, something that was not an option for her at her previous place of residence.

Freda has made several connections with other residents at Mei Domus, but she spends time reading to one particular resident. Freda sees herself as being more able than this resident and appears to enjoy providing some assistance to her, "I've made a lovely friend called Justine. I go and read to her. She's blind so at the moment I'm reading to her. I'm going Friday night actually." Freda reports that Mei Domus is friendly, open, and welcoming. She finds the other residents to be generally interesting and nice people. Freda sees herself as being someone who makes friends easily and developed friendships at her previous accommodation. She takes interest in other people and tries to find others who share some common interests such as cooking. However, she has not yet found anyone with similar interests. Although she talks about enjoying cooking, she has not engaged in any cooking since being at Mei Domus. The provision of meals by the staff inhibits her cooking for herself. She describes herself on a couple of occasions as being lazy in this regard and talks about no longer needing to cook as the staff does that for her. She justifies her lack of cooking by stating that if she were to cook as well as eating the meals prepared by the staff, she would "get fat and put on too much weight." As someone who was very active, her current inactivity impacts on the way she feels about herself.

Freda describes the staff at Mei Domus as being caring, lovely, and comments on the fact that she "hasn't met a crabby nurse yet." This is unlike her previous residence where she describes some of the staff as being "awful, they were horrible; they didn't offer to do anything for you." She describes how the staff at Mei Domus will regularly do small things for her like clean her glasses before giving them to her and, if she needs personal assistance, they are ready to offer help (for example, wiping her bottom if she has difficulty on the toilet). Freda sees this as very caring behavior. She believes that she is liked by the staff, which she attributes to her own good manners and behaviors. She states that,

> They make little comments to me, they'll often say to me, you're very easy to look after Freda. We all like looking after you because you're easy to [look after], you're very—congratulating of staff, because I thank them and I use my manners. They tell me that, so it's nice.

In contrast to her previous accommodation, Mei Domus provides Freda with room to move, space to put her things around her, "I can see all my things about and it's making me feel like myself again." It allows a level of independence, choice, and autonomy that was previously lacking. She experiences choice and flexibility in regard to the structure of her day at Mei Domus together with a sense of routine including regular physiotherapy appointments. There appears to be some imposed structure around meal times:

> Well, dinner is approximately about 12 or 12.15-ish. You can go at 12.30 if you like, but around that time you go down for your dinner. Same thing at night-time, dinner's around five, 5.15, 5.30-ish. If you go down then you should get your meal.

However, she still has choice regarding where she has her meals:

> You can have your meal in your room if you like. Sometimes I've had my meal in my room, I've been watching—sometimes in the afternoon I watch a bit of tennis on TV and it was a really good tennis game so I bought my meal back to my room so I could finish watching my tennis game. Yeah, you can have your meal in your room if you wish or you can have it in the dining room with everybody else. Do as you wish.

Freda has the sense that she can do as she wishes, there is a sense for her of being spoiled and well cared for: "The meals are tremendous, we're very spoilt. We have a very good cook and she gives us a wonderful selection of meals."

Although Mei Domus has exceeded Freda's expectations, it still did not constitute home. According to Freda, "There is no place like home." For her, home is a wonderful place, a place where her favorite meals are cooked by Mum. It is a place where she is with family, somewhere family can pop in with no restrictions, where she has her own things around her. Freda believes you can never replace home. Having her own things around her at Mei Domus is important to her and gives her a link to her past, her memories, providing her with history and identity: "They're [belongings] part of your past, part of your memories, you remember things, who gave them to you, when they gave them to you. They're just part of you." However, it is not enough just to have her things around her. Despite regular visits, her family is absent on a day-to-day basis, which makes it not-home: "My family aren't here all the time. Although my family do come to visit me and they come quite regularly, they're not here all the time." She misses the familiar experiences (for example, the cooking smells) that are associated with home. There are even positive things about Mei Domus that highlight the fact that is not her home. For instance, the large television in her apartment, which she enjoys, somehow reminds her that if she were at home she would not have such a large television.

Freda understands that she requires a high-level nursing and attendant care and is not in a position to live with her family. Mei Domus appears to be a good substitute for home; a place where she receives the care and direction she needs. Thus, in some ways, Mei Domus is providing the space for Freda to be herself again, to rebuild her postinjury self, which she differentiates from her preinjury self. She previously saw herself as a wife and mother, but she is no longer a wife and her role as a mother has changed dramatically. Some of this role change is a natural transition due to the age of her children; however, some of this change has been triggered by her need to change residence. The time spent in her previous residence created a distance between her and her children due to the restrictions imposed upon them:

> Well, what I was before I had my accident. I was a mother at home with three children to look after. I had a husband to consider. I don't have that here. I'm on my own here. Whereas when I was at home, I had three children and a husband to consider. I don't have them anymore. I miss my children, I miss them greatly. When I had my accident, my aneurysm, my daughter was only 10 years old, she was only a baby, so I miss having the children about. The two boys were a little bit older but they weren't much older. I've missed a lot of things with the kids.

Freda experiences Mei Domus as open and bright, a place where she can wander around and choose to spend time indoors or outside, she experiences the place as being beautiful. Despite the benefits of this environment, she would return to her family home if she could access the services she required. Home remains a place for Freda to go back to in future.

Therese

Therese is a female resident who was 52 years of age and has been married for 29 years. In 2002, like Freda, Therese had a brain aneurysm, which left her in a wheelchair. Prior to her aneurysm, Therese was a full-time mother to three children now aged between 17 and 20 years, a role from which she derived great pleasure. Following her aneurysm, Therese stayed in the hospital for two years and went home for the weekends. Therese's accommodation at the hospital was located with patients who had dementia.

When Therese initially moved to Mei Domus, she saw her family regularly. Her husband visited during the week with a friend of Therese's and again at the weekend with their children. They used to visit more frequently when Therese was in hospital; however she advised that the time there was very stressful and pressured. She describes Mei Domus as being calm and relaxed; a place where, "They make you feel wanted, so you really don't have any worries about that." Although Therese misses her family and telephones them daily, when they visit at Mei Domus, she feels a sense of pressure because she has got used to her "little unit—it's my little unit, my little den, I just like it here."

Access to her own telephone has allowed her to maintain regular contact with family and friends, her sister also contacts her from overseas weekly and is planning to come and stay with Therese. The option for people to stay at Mei Domus assists her in maintaining contact with others. Therese describes feeling relaxed and having more freedom now she is living at Mei Domus, which is not only positive for her but also the people in her life:

> I have more freedom here. I can talk to people, about the way I feel and everything. For a fact, my girlfriend came the other day, because I had a seizure at church and I couldn't make it to her place that night for dinner. She was worried and she came to see me. She was really happy to see I was so relaxed here. Then we went and had a cup of coffee downstairs. It's just like being at home. Everything is so relaxed.

For Therese, being at Mei Domus normalizes her disability; she has a sense of being accepted and welcomed, a sense of belonging that she no longer has within the community or even at her family home.

Over time, contact with her own family has reduced and Therese has formed relationships with other residents at Mei Domus and through these connections; she has the opportunity to spend time with another resident's child, which appears to fulfill a mother role for Therese:

> We just have a little chat at night. If I make a special meal, she'll [friend Barbie] come and help me and then we have dinner together sometimes here. It's really good . . . Even her little kid is really sweet. He chose this lounge as his bed. He comes, jumps on the lounge, puts the TV on and watches TV, because Barbie is busy doing her thing there, he treats this like his home. . . . It's lovely. He's like my kid, a big kid, a boy, a noisy boy.

The strongest relationships she appears to have made are with the staff at Mei Domus: "With the carers and nurses here, the friendship I've built up with them is so good. I really miss them when they are on holidays and stuff like that." Due to the relatively young age of the staff, her interactions with them provide further opportunities for mother-like experiences. Interestingly, she describes looking after the nurses like "they're my children, they're so young, they're good kids, they're really good people."

Therese has established some structure and routine for her days with assistance from the staff at Mei Domus who encourage her to be as independent as possible. This encouragement gives Therese a sense of pride, achievement, and independence,

> They don't force you to do anything and it's just, it's the way they tell you to do things. It's just a very nice way of rehab[ilitation]. They've got a nice way of doing rehab[ilitation] here. It's a beautiful way they do it. They make you feel you're wanted . . . Even yesterday [staff] got me to get a watering can. I felt so proud of myself and I went and filled the watering can full to the top from the bathroom and I was able to lift it. It was such a challenge and [staff] said, "You did it Therese, you did it. That's good, you can do it. If you did it once, you can do it again". Fantastic. That means I can do it every day.

Therese prefers now to think of Mei Domus as home, yet there appears to be some conflict in her mind. While she refers to Mei Domus as her home and has no desire to leave, she also does not want to be a burden to her family by returning home:

> To me, I prefer this as home—prefer to be here because if I go home I won't be welcome home. I'm a lot happier here. I know there's no restrictions here, I know I can press the bell, I don't feel bad to ask anyone, whereas if I go home there'd be things I need to ask for help and I'd feel restricted, because the kids are going to school and they

say, "oh Mum, we're busy, we've got no time." I don't think it's fair, that's why I prefer to be here. I think I'm being fair by them by staying in here.

To some extent, her decision is also based on her desire to take care of her own needs. Mei Domus provides a place where she feels wanted, relaxed, and safe. She has access to the therapies she needs, and she is comforted by knowing that there is staff to assist her when she requires. She acknowledges that this level of support would not be available if she moved back to her family home. However, she maintains the belief that, at some stage in the future when she is ready, she would like to return home:

> To me this is home. This will always be home. This is my home. I love this place. I love the people. I love the way it's set up . . . It's got room enough that the wheelchair can wheel around, you're not knocking things, and it's easy to get through. That's what's easy, whereas if I went home, to get through corners, half the time I was knocking through doors. It was a real pain . . . I feel very, very safe here and I know everyone, the carers are here to help me. They'll do everything possible, their best, to help me. Till I'm one hundred per cent sure that I'm fine to go home, I won't go home.

Although Therese has a sense of home at Mei Domus there is no real sense of permanence to this home. Staff members appear to provide some of the characteristics of family, but there is also a deep sense of loss in relation to her children.

Discussion

The similarities between Freda and Therese are clear in terms of demographics and experiences. They are the same age, both are mothers, both suffered an aneurysm, and have been living with their disability for the same length of time. Both moved to Mei Domus at a similar time (within six months of each other) and both had the experience of having to live in inappropriate accommodation prior to moving to Mei Domus. Although both have faced similar issues and experiences, the comparison of their stories demonstrates their vastly different ways of managing their experience and the impact this has had on their lives. So what is it that makes their experience of home different from each other?

This case study has demonstrated the comparative nature of home. It is an individual concept based on private memories and experiences. One's current home is experienced in relation to previous experiences of home and the extent to which it meets particular and unique requirements for building one's sense of comfort and belonging. Both women identified similar features of the sense of home, such as a place where they felt welcome, safe, and comfortable, and could make choices. Home was described as a space to have your own things, the ability to manipulate the environment to suit your own needs, with space and opportunity to develop and/or maintain deeper relationships with family and friends. Common features of the physical place, such as access to technology and a private telephone, assisted them to maintain contact with significant others. The ability to speak to loved ones and arrange visits without relying on staff to assist gave them a sense of freedom and choice, allowed them to maintain a sense of independence, and feel relaxed within their environment.

However, the interaction between home and family was critical to the distinction between the two women. For Therese, the presence of her family decreased her sense of home, but to compensate she had formed strong relationships with staff at Mei Domus. These relationships appeared to provide a substitute for family, allowing her to enact the highly desired mothering role due to the age difference between her and many of the young staff members. In contrast, Freda's experience of home was diminished by the absence of her family that could not be compensated for. For her, home is the place where family is always present. To account for the absence of her children, she compared Mei Domus to her childhood home with her own mother. This regression to her childhood experiences was defined by familiar cooking smells and favorite meals. Like Therese, Freda also perceived the staff as being friendly and caring. However, she did not seem to experience the same depth of relationship with staff. They did not appear to provide her with a substitute for family. For Freda, the longing to be with family remained strong and although she had regular visits from family, it was not enough to create a sense of home for Freda. It appeared that Therese was able to seek comfort through relationships with staff, whereas Freda sought comfort from the familiar memories and reminders of her real home.

The attitude and behavior of staff impacted on the residents' sense of home in both a positive and negative way. The way Therese was treated by staff and family created her sense of home. At Mei Domus, Therese felt encouraged by staff to increase her independence, for example, she had the opportunity and encouragement from staff to water her plants daily and do her washing up. She experienced staff members as patient and accepting of her disability, which contrasted with the experience of her own family, with whom she felt like a burden and believed they were ashamed of her disability. In contrast, Freda felt liked by the staff and welcome at Mei Domus, but her level of independence was negatively impacted by the intervention of staff in everyday tasks, such as cooking.

The quality of relationships with staff clearly impacted on relationships with their family, which then influenced their sense of belonging and home at Mei Domus. When the experience of relating with staff was highly positive and informal relationships were formed, the connection with staff added to the sense of home within the residential environment, in many ways substituting for family contact. In contrast, when staff relationships were experienced as positive, but remained formal, the absence of family became even more apparent, serving as a reminder that the residence was not home. It is therefore important that the family situation and responses of each individual resident in absence of family are understood by staff and facilitated in the most appropriate manner.

The physical environment also impacted on the residents' sense of comfort and belonging. The space and layout of the environment allowed ease of movement, and choice about where and with whom they spent their time. Therese compared this to her experience at her family home where she had difficulty maneuvering around the space, constantly bumping into walls and doorways. The accessibility of Mei Domus created a more relaxed space for her in which she could feel at home. However, when aspects of the environment create difficulties for the residents (e.g., spaces prevent them from managing small tasks themselves, such as making a cup of tea), or tasks were routinely carried out by staff, their reliance on staff was increased, highlighting their disability and impacting negatively on their sense of independence and identity. Thus, it could be tentatively concluded that place, people, and personal expectations interact to create a sense of home for residents. The ability to make choices and develop an acceptable level of independence combines with these other features to create a sense of belonging and a connection to a physical place that can enable it to be thought of as home.

In conclusion, it is the physical environment and the residents' ability and opportunity to have choice, independence, and a sense of freedom; and the relationships experienced within that environment, whether they be with family, friends, or staff, that interact to create a sense of home. The space and opportunity to spend unrestricted time with family and friends and engage in more natural and individual daily routines has a positive influence on the residents' sense of belonging and is therefore an important consideration for any future residential environments. However, while a place can provide a person with the basic needs and comforts and a sense of security, it cannot replace the self-generated sense of home that comes with family. It may be able to mirror some aspects of that home, but the experience of home is diminished when important people are not around at all times. For some people though, it does appear that relationships with staff can provide a substitute familial experience and this ought to be managed within the context of paid relationships. Many features combine to create the sense of home for an individual, and this expose of two individuals with brain injury living in a residential care environment has highlighted the importance of critical relationships (i.e., family and care staff) and the process of engagement within the home environment. Further, the feeling of non-home, as experienced when the characteristic physical and relational features of home are absent, highlights the threat of *unintended institutionalization* within these purpose-built environments. Overall, findings from this qualitative investigation bring new meaning and consequence to the concept of the family home.

References

Annison, J. E. (2000). Towards a clearer understanding of the meaning of "home." *Journal of Intellectual & Developmental Disability, 25*(4), 251–262.

Dyck, I., Kontos, P., Angus, J., & McKeever, P. (2005). The home as a site for long-term care: Meanings and management of bodies and spaces. *Health & Place, 11*(2), 173–185.

Maslow, A. H. (1943). A theory of human motivation. *Psychological Review, 50*(4), 370–396.

Muenchberger, H., Ehrlich, C., Kendall, E., & Vit, M. (2012). Experience of place for young adults under 65 years with complex disabilities moving into purpose-built residential care. *Social Science & Medicine, 75*(12), 2151–2159. Ridgway, P., Simpson, A., Wittman, F. D., & Wheeler, G. (1994). Homemaking and the community building: Notes on empowerment and place. *Journal of Mental Health Administration, 21*(4), 407–418.

Ruddick, W. (1995). Transforming homes into hospitals. In: Arras, J. D. (Ed.), *Bringing the hospital home* (pp. 166–179). Baltimore, MD: John Hopkins University Press..

Stedman, R. C. (2002). Toward a social psychology of place: Predicting behavior from place-based cognitions, attitude, and identity. *Environment and Behavior, 34*(5), 561–581.

Tamm, M. (1999). What does a home mean and when does it cease to be a home? *Disability and Rehabilitation, 21*, 49–55.

Tuan, Y. F. (1977). *Space and place: the perspective of experience*. Minneapolis: University of Minnesota Press.

CHAPTER 13

The International Community-based Rehabilitation Model: A Way of Assisting People with Brain Injuries, Their Families, and Communities

Pim Kuipers, Susan Gauld, Melissa Kendall, Sharon Smith, and Russell Bowen

For 80 percent of people with disabilities in the world (specifically those in developing countries), there are few formal services. Indeed, of the more than one billion disabled people living in developing countries, the majority of services we take for granted in economically developed countries, simply do not exist. In these countries formal rehabilitation, employment, and independence services, policies, laws, technologies, aids, appliances, and equipment, which contribute to quality of life and well-being, are not available. The community-based rehabilitation (CBR) model was first promoted by the World Health Organization (WHO) in the mid-1970s to respond to people with disabilities in developing countries (Turmusani, Vreede, & Wirz, 2002). CBR was designed to address the limited nature of the rehabilitation workforce in developing countries through the provision of basic community services at a community level. Incorporating principles of primary health care (PHC) and relevant rehabilitation practices, the model sought to use local resources and build local skills (Hartley, Finkenflugel, Kuipers, & Thomas, 2009) to assist people with disabilities. The CBR approach is the primary means by which people with disabilities in most countries of the world have had any access to rehabilitation or disability services (Evans, Zinkin, Harpham, & Chaudury, 2001). The most widely used definition of CBR is

A strategy within general community development for the rehabilitation, equalization of opportunities, and social inclusion of all people with disabilities . . . implemented through the combined efforts of people with disabilities themselves, their families and communities, and the appropriate health, education, vocational, and social services. (ILO, UNESCO, & WHO, 2004, p.2)

However, one of the defining characteristics of CBR is that it continues to evolve. Initially CBR approaches tended to focus on disability alone, sometimes failing to recognize the disabling effects of the social and physical environments, and the limited engagement of people with disabilities in community life. However, contemporary approaches to CBR are more strongly focused on building the participation of people with disabilities in the life and work of their communities and societies. CBR initiatives increasingly focus on the community, community organizations, and the role they play in bringing about greater participation of persons with disabilities in all spheres of life. Internationally CBR agencies are increasingly promoting an inclusive development agenda, seeking the active engagement of people with disabilities across numerous sectors (WHO, UNESCO, ILO, & IDDC, 2010). Proponents emphasize a human rights approach to disability and rehabilitation (WHO et al., 2010), and foster community engagement in disability issues (Kuipers & Harknett, 2008). Increasingly however, the strengths and potential of this approach are being recognized in economically developed countries (Kendall, Muenchberger, & Catalano, 2009), specifically to assist people with acquired brain injury (ABI) (Doig, Fleming, Cornwell, & Kuipers, 2009). However, because of the general nature of CBR, initiatives tend not to be disability-specific, so services targeted directly to people with traumatic or acquired brain injuries are not common.

CBR is usually conducted or provided in natural community settings such as the person's home, rather than formal service delivery settings such as hospital or center-based environments. The active engagement of people with disabilities, family, and even community members in service delivery is core to CBR. People with disabilities are viewed as partners in, if not active directors of, the process (Kuipers & Doig, 2011). As a strategy, CBR seeks to equip, empower, and educate people with disabilities and all stakeholders toward the end goals of greater independence, more community participation, and increased quality of life (WHO et al., 2010). CBR typically seeks to assist people with disabilities to actively contribute to their own communities. Importantly, it also encourages community members to promote and respect human rights, to maximize accessibility to resources, and to build opportunities for participation (WHO et al., 2010). In CBR, skill transfer to the community and systemic change are considered important aspirations. CBR programs are likely to be aimed at achieving broader social and systemic changes as well as maximizing social inclusion and improvements in individuals' functional capacity (Kuipers & Doig, 2011).

As may be expected, the international CBR model does not typically address early impairment or disability in the acute stages of injury or illness. In most cases, the approach assists people whose impairments and disabilities require long term rehabilitation and care (Kuipers & Doig, 2011). The exact nature of CBR services depends on the needs of the particular person or persons within their context, the presence of disability supports in the family and community, the existence of environmental resources (including availability of generic services such as community health services), the availability of skills and expertise, practical feasibility, and the availability of funding.

Internationally, family members play a vital role in CBR. These family members and community volunteers may only be provided with basic training, but rely on their community knowledge. They are often supported by a local committee. In some cases volunteers are assisted by intermediate-level voluntary workers, with limited access to qualified health and rehabilitation professionals. CBR workers rarely work in discipline-specific roles, but tend to take on more generic tasks akin to rehabilitation coordinators or case managers. CBR workers often facilitate and organize a person's rehabilitation in the community and promote communication and coordination between the person with a disability, their family, health and community services, and all stakeholders involved in the person's life.

A key strength of the international CBR model is the enhanced opportunity for specific education for family members, support workers, or health care workers, and more general skill-sharing across family, friends, work colleagues, community members, and others who may be informally supporting the person. As a result, family members are likely to be directly involved in rehabilitation. Furthermore, the approach is likely to be more collaborative, engage work colleagues, community members, and extended family who may be in a position to help the person achieve their goals. Indeed, the core mechanism of CBR is collaboration: the development of strong relationships between families, communities, people with disabilities and the appropriate health, education, vocational, and social services. These characteristics of family engagement, collaboration, and community integration are highly desired yet elusive in many Western rehabilitation programs.

Future Challenges for Community-based Rehabilitation

The transfer of skills to people with disabilities, family, and community members is central to the international CBR model. How this is best achieved is a question that requires greater attention. Specifically, there is a need for a shift in the roles and functions of health professionals to enable them to take on more strategic roles and facilitate more empowering strategies in CBR (Lang, 2011). However, such a shift will require a more rights-based approach to the training of health professionals, in addition to one based on clinical expertise.

Other critical challenges in CBR include: sustaining relationships between rehabilitation professionals and people with disabilities, enhancing networks and partnerships (especially between disabled people's organizations and governments), building greater connections in communities and increasingly building partnerships with industry and private enterprise (Kuipers & Doig, 2011). The philosophy of empowerment is central to CBR, which requires a shift in thinking of health professionals from being expert toward being facilitators and partners.

There is increasing interest in CBR theory, interventions, outcomes, and evidence, reflected in calls for improvement in the rigor and reporting of CBR in research and project evaluations (Finkenflugel, Cornielje, & Velema, 2007), and the use of more innovative research methods (Kuipers, Wirz, & Hartley, 2008). The evolutionary nature of CBR and its responsiveness to critiques is reflected in the new CBR guidelines and matrix (WHO et al., 2010), which emphasize the human rights-based elements of CBR. The CBR model is now ready to be examined more rigorously, applied more consistently, and integrated more effectively into national and international policy making. Although its application in developing countries is established, the potential for greater implementation in economically developed countries remains a challenge.

Community Rehabilitation in Economically Developed Countries

The interest in community rehabilitation in economically developed countries can be related to gradual shifts in philosophical perspective, practical considerations, financial constraints, and preferences of people with disabilities (Kuipers & Doig, 2011). It is also a function of demographic changes (e.g., aging population), service changes (e.g., reduction of hospital lengths of stay), illness trajectory factors (e.g., enhanced survival after serious injury), as well as a recognition that community services can deliver comparable outcomes (Barnes & Radermacher, 2001; Langhorne et al., 2005; Doig, Fleming, Kuipers, & Cornwell, 2010). Alongside this shift has been an increase in the availability and the use of a range of services in the broader community. For example, for people who are aging, services such as meal delivery, community nursing, respite services, and domestic assistance are increasingly becoming available in local communities.

If CBR is to have substantial impact on economically developed countries, where rehabilitation is often provided according to diagnostic groupings, it will require strategies to engage and inform communities on disability-specific issues, as well as flexibility on the part of providers. Most importantly, the implementation of CBR in economically developed countries requires viable community-based implementation processes and strategies.

In contrast to the international model, many rehabilitation programs in economically developed countries while physically located in local communities, exhibit few of the collaborative and community-focused dimensions that characterize CBR internationally. A key review of community programs for people with brain injuries in economically developed countries identified six types of community programs including home-based behavior management, outdoor experiential education programs, client/carer educational training, community-based peer support, interdisciplinary team building programs, and telephone counseling (Evans & Brewis, 2008). However, none of these focused on engaging with local communities, as in the international CBR approach.

An Example: Instigating CBR in an Economically Developed Context

Over the years, a few community initiatives have been instigated in economically developed countries to support people with ABI. One innovative example, which trialed a CBR approach, was a two-year project undertaken in collaboration with two Indigenous /Aboriginal communities in Cape York, far north Queensland, Australia, by a state-wide service for adults who have ABI (Gauld, Smith, & Kendall, 2011). Some of the unique challenges of instigating CBR in these contexts are described below.

In Australia, the incidence of brain injuries among Indigenous people is up to four times the rate of that in non-Indigenous populations (Kendall & Marshall, 2004). Indigenous people, particularly Indigenous women, are disproportionately represented in hospitalizations for brain injury due to assaults, with the rate amongst Indigenous people being 21 times higher than that for non-Indigenous people (Jamieson, Harrison, & Berry, 2008).

In keeping with CBR principles, the Cape York project relied heavily on consultation with communities, including key health and disability stakeholders, service providers, individuals with brain injury, their families, and interested community members. The commitment to and process of consultation was greatly assisted by the employment of a local worker in each community. Working closely with a designated community member facilitated the development of close working relationships within each community.

The project relied on participatory action research (PAR) to explore how ABI and the resultant disability was perceived by members of the two Aboriginal and/or Torres Strait Islander communities, and identifying the ongoing needs and existing supports of people with ABI and their families in these communities. This method was chosen to maximize community consultation, build engagement, and ensure that the project resulted in outcomes for each community and for people with ABI. Participatory approaches are advocated to most accurately reflect the experiences of marginalized, rural, remote, and Aboriginal communities (Minore, Boone, Katt, Kinch, & Burke, 2004), and are highly consistent with involving people with disabilities and communities in the planning and development of CBR services (Kuipers, Kendall, & Hancock, 2001). The essential elements of PAR are collaboration, participation, and reflection, which take place during repeated cycles of planning, acting, and review (Stringer, 1996). The planning cycles involve extensive formal and documented discussion regarding perceived problems and necessary actions through individual interviews, small groups, and focus groups. The dynamic parts involve the researchers and participants implementing actions, whilst the review cycles involve assessment of actions through collected information (Gauld, Smith, & Kendall, 2011).

The process of engaging with communities was facilitated by an expert advisory group made up of representatives from the relevant Aboriginal and Torres Strait Islander health agency, the disability sector, the academic sector, and a family member. This group facilitated contact with communities across the state, inviting participation in the project. The methodology allowed communities to self-select, depending on whether brain injury was seen as a priority by at least some community members.

Two remote communities indicated an interest in this project, resulting in initial visits to these communities to discuss the project in more depth. Both communities agreed to proceed, and after ethics committee approval, consultation with community members commenced through individual and group interviews, focus groups, and informal discussion (Gauld, Smith, & Kendall, 2011).

Consultations were based on questions around the local perception of brain injury, the needs of people with brain injuries and their families, the supports available and currently used, as well as barriers to support. From these consultations, planning for the project could begin. One community responded well to organized community meetings and information sessions, but in the other community, individual or small group consultations proved more successful. The process of regularly reviewing actions and planning future actions occurred through verbal feedback, often following presentation of a new development or plan. For example, one community produced posters about brain injury prevention using local language. When these posters were presented at a meeting, constructive feedback resulted in appropriate modifications. These discussions with community members and key stakeholders enabled agreement to proceed and new suggestions for action. Thus the project evolved over a natural course, as directed by each community.

The process used by Gauld and colleagues (Gauld, Smith, & Kendall, 2011), also determined who within communities became involved. Key stakeholders identified themselves within the process of planning, action-ing, and reviewing. Recognizing the importance of the broader social and service context of communities, other community members, key commu-nity groups, local services, and other stakeholders were also regularly consulted. These included justice groups, home and community care ser-vices, primary health clinics, disability services (Queensland Department of Communities), and other visiting services (e.g., Royal Flying Doctor Service and Far North Queensland Division of Rural General Practice), as well as individuals with brain injury, their families, and other community members who regularly attended meetings or made themselves available to the project staff for consultation and review of plans and actions.

Employment of Local Community-based Rehabilitation Worker

The selection of the local CBR worker was another outcome of this con-sultation process (Gauld, Smith, & Kendall, 2011). The employment of local brain injury workers is consistent with CBR principles as well as with the principles of cultural safety. Recognizing that Indigenous peo-ple typically feel more comfortable relating to another Indigenous person is an approach that promotes cultural safety, fostering "an environment where clients, families and community members have health care choices and their values and attitudes respected" (NRHA, 2006).

A critical role of this local worker in each community was to assist with contacts, advise on cultural and community protocols, organize inter-views/meetings, gather and review information as well as taking a lead role in assisting in consultations with members of the communities and actioning the plans made by the communities. The local worker provided a key to successful community engagement and consultation, and was evidence of a commitment to this process. Employment of a local worker in each community was achieved early in the project, and with relative ease, despite some initial doubt among a few community members that an untrained local person would be able to fulfill the tasks.

According to Gauld and colleagues (2011), workers in both communi-ties displayed genuine enthusiasm for the issue of brain injury and were willing to work closely with all involved in the project to promote activi-ties within each community. Both workers were proactive in suggesting activities that educate the community about brain injury. Initially, local workers assisted the project team in consulting with the community and engaging in education, rehabilitation, and consultation sessions within the community. However, the roles of the local workers evolved over time, with some differences between the two communities emerging due to the localized nature of the process. In one community the focus became education of the whole community about brain injury prevention and how to assist someone who has a brain injury. In the second community, individuals with brain injury were referred for services, with the local worker having a more direct role in the provision of support. Interestingly, final consultations in this community revealed difficulties for the worker due to the limited support available. Suggestions made by the community to address this isolation and lack of support included a mentoring system, akin to a CBR committee, which was trialed.

Specific Challenges in Implementing a Community-based Rehabilitation-type Model

The participatory CBR approach was critical to the outcomes achieved in both communities, but it did pose problems in the early stages of the project. Understandably, people wanted to know more about the project and its outcomes before agreeing to participate. However, this was not possible within a locally responsive approach in which the outcomes are only determined through the course of the initiative. Cultural and language differences were also highlighted particularly through the provision of information about the project and brain injury. Adapting content so that it meaningfully reflected the culture and context of these two communities was necessary for the successful transfer of knowledge. There was a need to balance medical and professional terms with the literacy and educational levels of people within communities and of the CBR workers.

The project team in the Gauld et al. (2011) study was aware that developing working relationships with individuals within each community would be time-consuming and would require a building of trust. The consistency of workers, the commitment to follow through on decisions made, and the engagement of local people were the key elements for trust to develop. It was imperative to stay focused on the agreed strategy and allow the process to develop in a timely fashion.

The commitment to consultation with people with brain injury and their families proved challenging at times. From stories told to the project team, it appeared that many cases of brain injury had not been formally diagnosed. Not surprisingly, some people did not want to identify that they had a brain injury, as they felt they were getting on with their lives, and had recovered from their injury. People were also reluctant to tell their personal stories to outsiders. Thus, consultation began with those who were willing to participate, and broader consultation became possible over time, as people developed trust and became more aware of the project.

Initial consultations revealed that there was considerable misunderstanding about brain injury, and often confusion with mental health problems. Therefore, communities and services initially needed sufficient information so they could identify aspects of brain injury. The community education requested by the communities continued to focus on this issue so, over time, people's understanding of brain injury increased significantly. The communities also created opportunities for local people to voluntarily share their stories of brain injury during community meet-ings or education sessions, indicating the degree of community engage-ment, and the priority placed on local knowledge and experience.

Initial interviews and focus groups indicated that local stakeholders often resent the demands created by visiting and outreach models of re-habilitation services used in many rural and remote areas. In contrast, using a CBR approach, this project sought to foster local community lead-ership that engaged and consulted with many community services. It was also responsive to each context. In keeping with a CBR focus on capacity-building, it was necessary to approach the two communities in ways that minimized the burden on them and supported their existing service arrangements. This approach contrasted with the challenges inherent in some other visiting services.

The project recognized that interest levels and availability of com-munity members fluctuated over the life of the project and were depen-dent on other events occurring in the community or within families over time. Open communication with key stakeholders and the local workers in each community provided information on preferred timing of visits for maximum benefit to the community and generally allowed plans to change accordingly. In Indigenous communities in particular, flexibility, open communication, and awareness of people's commitments (personal, ceremonial/cultural and community) are critical for successful engage-ment of people with ABI, family members, and others.

Formal ABI rehabilitation and outreach services may have difficulty providing the degree of consultation outlined here, and may recognize that the financial, time, and practical aspects of travelling to remote com-munities can be difficult to sustain. In a community-based approach, ac-commodating competing demands and exercising sensitivity to people's ability to attend to project priorities must take a longer term view so that relationships are strengthened, allowing longer term outcomes to occur.

Reflections on Implementing Community-based Rehabilitation in an Economically Developed Context

Overall, this chapter has explored the use of the international CBR model in Indigenous communities in Australia and has demonstrated how it can be applied to ABI. The PAR method used to implement this CBR project described above maximized community consultation, engagement, and outcomes for people with ABI living in these remote communities. Whilst there were obvious challenges in the process, the project was success-ful in moving from consultations to actions. Employment of a local CBR worker was imperative in facilitating this process. CBR is a tailored and flexible approach that seeks to support the rights and choice of people with disabilities. Hallmarks of the CBR model are that it is strongly com-munity focused, and that it involves the community in deciding on the direction of interventions, and the delivery of services. The active role of local people throughout the process is central, particularly local people with disabilities. While it may also be resource-intensive and time-extensive, given the social, community, and service barriers that people with brain injuries face, the potential benefit of such an approach for these people, their families, and communities is substantial.

References

Barnes, M. P., & Radermacher, H. (2001). Neurological rehabilitation in the community. *Journal of Rehabilitation Medicine, 33*(6), 244–248.

Doig, E., Fleming, J., Cornwell, P. L., & Kuipers, P. (2009). Qualitative exploration of a client-centered, goal-directed approach to community-based occupational therapy for adults with traumatic brain injury. *American Journal of Occupational Therapy, 63*(5), 559–568.

Doig, E., Fleming, J., Kuipers, P., & Cornwell, P. (2010). Comparison of rehabilitation outcomes in day hospital and home settings for people with acquired brain injury—a systematic review. *Disability and Rehabilitation 32*(25), 2061–2077.

Evans, L., & Brewis, C. (2008). The efficacy of community-based rehabilitation programmes for adults with TBI. *International Journal of Therapy and Rehabilitation 15*(10), 446–458.

Evans, P. J., Zinkin, P., Harpham, T., & Chaudury, G. (2001). Evaluation of community-based rehabilitation for disabled persons in developing countries. *Social Science & Medicine, 53*(3), 333–348.

Finkenflugel, H., Cornielje, H., & Velema, J. (2007). The use of classification models in the evaluation of CBR programmes. *Disability and Rehabilitation, 30*(5), 348–354.

Gauld, S., Smith, S., & Kendall, M. B. (2011). Using participatory action research in community-based rehabilitation for people with acquired brain injury: From service provision to partnership with Aboriginal communities. *Disability and Rehabilitation, 33*(19–20), 1901–1911.

Hartley, S., Finkenflugel, H., Kuipers, P., & Thomas, M. (2009). Community-based rehabilitation: Opportunity and challenge. *Lancet, 374*(9704), 1803–1804.

International Labour Office (ILO), United Nations Educational, Scientific and Cultural Organization (UNESCO), & World Health Organization (WHO). (2004). *Joint position paper—CBR: A strategy for rehabilitation, equalization of opportunities, poverty reduction and social inclusion of people with disabilities.* Geneva, Switzerland: World Health Organisation.

Jamieson, L. M., Harrison, J., & Berry, J. G. (2008). Hospitalisation for head injury due to assault among Indigenous and non-Indigenous Australians, July 1999–June 2005. *Medical Journal of Australia, 188*(10), 576–579.

Kendall, E., & Marshall, C. A. (2004). Factors that prevent equitable access to rehabilitation for Aboriginal Australians with disabilities: The need for culturally safe rehabilitation. *Rehabilitation Psychology, 49*(1), 5–13.

Kendall, E., Muenchberger, H., & Catalano, T. (2009). The move towards community-based rehabilitation in industrialised countries: Are we equipped for the challenge? *Disability & Rehabilitation, 31*(26), 2164–2173.

Kuipers, P., & Doig, E. (2011). Community Based Rehabilitation. In J. Stone & M. Blouin (Series Ed.), *International encyclopedia of rehabilitation,* Buffalo, NY: CIRRIE. Retrieved from http://cirrie.buffalo.edu/encyclopedia/en/article/362/

Kuipers, P., & Harknett, S. (2008). Considerations in the quest for evidence in community based rehabilitation. *Asia Pacific Disability Rehabilitation Journal, 19*(2), 3–14.

Kuipers, P., Kendall, E., & Hancock, T. (2001). Developing a rural community-based disability service: (I) Service framework and implementation strategy. *Australian Journal of Rural Health, 9*(1), 22–28.

Kuipers, P., Wirz, S., & Hartley, S. (2008). Systematic synthesis of community-based rehabilitation (CBR) project evaluation reports for evidence-based policy: a proof-of-concept study. *BMC International Health and Human Rights, 8*(3), 1–15.

Lang, R. (2011). Community-based rehabilitation and health professional practice: Developmental opportunities and challenges in the global North and South. *Disability & Rehabilitation, 33*(2), 165–173.

Langhorne, P., Taylor, G., Murray, G., Dennis, M., Anderson, C., Bautz-Holter, E. . . . Wolfe, C. (2005). Early supported discharge services for stroke patients: a meta-analysis of individual patients' data. *The Lancet, 365*(9458), 501–506.

Minore, B., Boone, M., Katt, M., Kinch, P., & Birch, S. (2004). Addressing the realities of health care in northern aboriginal communities through participatory action research. *Journal of Interprofessional Care, 18*(4), 360–368.

National Rural Health Alliance (NRHA). (2006). *Position paper—Aboriginal and Torres Strait Islander health workers.* Canberra, Australian Capital Territory: National Rural Health Alliance.

Stringer, E. (1996). *Action research: a handbook for practitioners.* Thousand Oaks, CA: Sage.

Turmusani, M., Vreede, A., & Wirz, S. L. (2002). Some ethical issues in community-based rehabilitation initiatives in developing countries. *Disability and Rehabilitation, 24*(10), 558–564.

World Health Organisation (WHO), United Nations Educational, Scientific and Cultural Organization (UNESCO), International Labour Office (ILO), & International Disability Development Consortium (IDDC). (2010). *Introductory booklet—Community-based rehabilitation CBR guidelines: Towards community-based inclusive development.* Geneva: World Health Organisation Press.

CHAPTER 14

Culture, Disability, and Caregiving for People with Traumatic Brain Injury

Paul Leung

The phone call for assistance came from an insurance company almost at wit's end about what to do with a 30-something Chinese American chef who had sustained a traumatic brain injury (TBI) almost two years earlier. The chef was living with his brother and sister-in-law in a small Midwestern community where he had worked in a Chinese restaurant. After the accident, initial hospitalization and several months of rehabilitation, the sister-in-law assumed the role of primary caretaker although her brother-in-law was probably able to take care of many of his own needs. The insurance case manager believed that the chef was able to go back to work. However, the family, and especially the sister-in-law insisted that he was ill and needed care.

This example illustrates the sometimes complex and often frustrating task of working at the intersection of disability, culture, ethnicity, and caregiving. In this case, reality conflicted with perceptions of ability, beliefs about what constitutes disability, and role expectations for caregiving. Differences of opinion and interpretations about disability after TBI had to be resolved to break the stalemate. Ethnicity and culture were significant variables that affected the outcome. The chef obviously had some residual functional limitations that affected his capacity to care for himself, but more importantly, in his familial context, he was perceived as being sick and needing continuing care and support.

Similar situations occur every day and will undoubtedly continue to increase in American society in the years ahead as America's population continues to diversify. The Family Caregiver Alliance, an organization devoted to needs of families who provide care at home, pointed out in a recent report that caregiving "will preoccupy American families well into the 21st century" (Feinberg, Gray, & Kelly, 2002, p. 4). The American Association of Retired Persons (AARP) national survey on caregiving in the United States suggested that caregiving will become a "prevalent and a normative experience" (AARP, 2004, p. 3). A more recent AARP survey (AARP, 2009) estimated that 22 percent of people will provide care each year for one or more ill or disabled family members or friends of all ages.

The focus of this chapter is on caregiving and disability following TBI within the context of ethnicity and culture. Although this chapter refers to the U.S. context, the combination of culture and caregiving is also important in other countries. Additionally, much of what is known about caregiving following TBI is generalized from a broader caregiving perspective. Emerging populations with a dominant Western culture often have different values and traditions from the white middle class majority. Consequently there will be an increasing global need to understand disability, ethnicity, and culture, and the impact of these factors on caregiving. The task of exploring this intersection following TBI is daunting and complex. This chapter highlights the general lack of knowledge about the role of ethnicity and culture on caregiving for persons with traumatic brain injury. This chapter also provides a framework for further exploration of the impact ethnicity may have on the caregiving process.

Caregiving for people with TBI who are from diverse backgrounds is becoming more important as our population continues to age and as medical and technological advances add to survival and life span following brain injury. Caregiving has received increasing attention during the last few years in the United States as the cost of health and medical services increase. Caregiving has been defined as providing "unpaid care to a relative or friend. . . . to help them take care of themselves" (Wagner, 1997, p. 3). Two broad categorizations of caregiving are instrumental and expressive (Wood & Wan, 1992) caregiving. Instrumental caregiving involves assistance with personal care functions and activities of daily living whereas expressive caregiving involves sharing in social activities, emotional support, and just being there (Wood & Wan, 1992).

An estimated 4.1 million people aged between 21 and 64 need personal assistance and 6.8 million people aged 65 or older have mobility and self-care limitations. Further, an estimated 30 million people discharged from hospitals need post–acute care assistance each year (NINR, 2001). Within these groups, those categorized as ethnic often have more complex health needs, less support, and greater need for caregiving than white middle class populations (Bethell & Lansky, 2001; Collins et al., 2002).

The WHO International Classification of Functioning, Disability, and Health (ICF) mandates an understanding of the context in which functioning occurs as an inherent part of the definition of disability. Thus, "a person's functioning and disability is conceived as the dynamic inter-action between health conditions and contextual factors" (WHO, 2000, p. 10). Definitions and descriptions of disability should take into account whether or not a condition is perceived as disabling by the individual and family. Of course, the perception or nonperception of disability is likely to be interpreted within the cultural or ethnic milieu in which the individual or family lives, making ethnicity inherent in considerations about disability.

Translations from languages other than English complicate what is meant by disability or what is disabling. Differences in world views or perspectives may depend on the extent to which an individual or family adheres to the traditions and culture of their origin, or how much that individual or family has become acculturated or even assimilated into mainstream U.S. culture, the primary language used in communication and how that individual and family view their identity. Geographic isolation from others of the same ethnic/racial background may also play a role. An American family of Chinese descent living in a small Midwestern community where no other Asian families live provides a vastly different milieu from that of a similar Chinese American family living in southern California in an enclave such as Monterey Park. In considering the impact of cultural context on disability, all these variants need to be explored.

Culture Defined

Culture is defined as the sum total of the values, beliefs, rules, and practices of a group including commonly used customs, communication systems, as well as artifacts produced or used by the group (Rosenthal, 1986; Sue DW & Sue D, 2002; Valle, 1998). Culture refers to "the shared, and largely learned, attributes of a group of people" (U.S. Surgeon General, 2002, p. 9). The U.S. Surgeon General's (2002) definition of culture emphasized the need for caution regarding the assumptions of shared culture:

> People who are placed, either by census categories or through self-identification, into the same racial or ethnic group are often assumed to share the same culture. Yet this assumption is an overgeneralization because not all members grouped together in a given category will share the same culture (p. 9).

It is also important to note that culture is not static, but is a changing and evolving process.

In summing up the complexity of culture, the Surgeon General noted, "Immigrants from different parts of the world arrive in the United States with their own culture but gradually begin to adapt." The term acculturation refers to the socialization process by which minority groups gradually learn and adopt selective elements of the dominant culture. Yet that dominant culture is itself transformed by its interaction with minority groups. Making matters more complex, the immigrant group may form its own subculture, distinct from both its country of origin and the dominant culture. The Chinatowns of major cities in the United States often exemplify the blending of Chinese traditions and the American context (U.S. Surgeon General, 2002, p. 9). Thus culture, while seemingly simple to define, embraces so many different aspects of life that its impact on daily life is profound. These relationships between culture, disability, and caregiving are particularly difficult to isolate and describe.

Culture and Caregiving

The cornerstone of current U.S. disability policy focuses on choice, independence, and integration or inclusion in the community for persons with disabilities. However, within this context, the "vast majority of direct care (about 64%) is provided by families, friends, and neighbors" (U.S. Department of Health and Human Services, 2002, p. 13). In other words, there is a systemic assumption that direct care necessitated by disability is the responsibility of family rather than government. Government policies related to caregiving and disability range widely, but often there is no formal policy or resources allocated. Caregiving by families usually occurs because there are few other options available to them. The absence of specific policy means that families, and especially families from ethnic groups, are forced to provide their own care for any family members who have disabilities.

Although culture may dictate "how to be healthy, how to behave when ill, how to care, and how to cure" (Pask, 2000, p. 12), there is a pressing need for cross-cultural research on caregiving. Young and Kahana (1995) described a conceptual model that offers some potential for exploring issues of ethnicity and caregiving, but there is very limited use of such models. Although the significance of culture to the caregiving process seems logical, the historical response of human service programs has been to assume that American culture is homogeneous and synonymous with white middle class values and beliefs. Clients or consumers are expected to adjust their needs to those addressed by the programs that are offered (Valle, 1998). Little empirical knowledge is available about caregiving for persons with disabilities in the context of ethnicity and culture. Although unknown, the burden of caregiving may be greater for non-white families than for white families. Tennstedt and Chang (1998) investigated differences in the need for and receipt of informal care among a range of groups in northeastern United States and found that ethnicity played an important role in explaining the findings.

The prevalence of caregiving among different ethnic populations related to disability following traumatic brain injury is unknown. Most surveys related to caregiving focus on specific groups, such as people aged 50 and older or children, rather than specific disability groups. The AARP survey (2004) found that the prevalence of caregiving for the elderly was higher among Asian (31.7%) and African American (29.4%) households than among Hispanic (26.8%) or white (24%) households. However, there is a generally higher incidence and prevalence of disability within ethnic populations, so it would be expected that there would be more need for caregiving (National Council on Disability, 1993; Smart J & Smart DW, 1997). For example, 75 percent of Hispanic American and 60 percent of African American people with mental illness live at home with their families in contrast to one-third of European American families (Lefley, 1996). Lefley (1996) further indicated that Hispanic and Asian families were more likely than other groups to keep a family member with a mental illness at home. African American elderly are more likely than white elderly to live in an extended family household (Angel & Tienda, 1982). Cantor, Gelfand, and Kutzik (1979) reported higher levels of support among Hispanic families than either white or African American families. Lubben, Becerra, Gelfand, and Barressi (1987) found that Hispanic families were more likely to help elderly family members and that the extended family remained "one of the most structural components of Hispanic culture" (p. 130). In terms of the impact of caregiving, African American and Hispanic caregivers report less sense of seclusion than white caregivers (Cox, Monk, Barresi, & Stull, 1993). Hispanic caregivers depend more on formal services for assistance than African Americans (Cox et al., 1993). Ethnicity may have both positive and negative influences on how caregiving is perceived (Young & Kahana, 1995).

In one study, Hispanic people and black non-Hispanic people were more likely than white non-Hispanic people to need help with personal care from another person (Ory, Hoffman, Yee, Tennstedt, & Schultz, 1999). Less is known about the experience of Asian Americans and Pacific Islanders because data is insufficient to represent groups that are relatively small in number. Navaie-Waliser et al. (2001) found that 70 percent of caregivers received no formal assistance. Navaie-Waliser and colleagues (2001) also reported that black caregivers were more likely to have unmet needs than white caregivers. A recent AARP survey (2001) of multicultural baby boomers, who have been called the sandwich generation, highlighted differences among ethnic groups. For example, Hispanic American families reported the heaviest caregiving role and also expended more effort to care for their family members than some other groups. Asian American families most often confessed guilt for not doing more caregiving and were also most likely to indicate that they experienced stress as result of caring for family members. African Americans, more than any other group, included siblings as part of their definition of immediate family. The significance of informal caregiving or support in this latter culture may stem from the many decades during which they were isolated from mainstream health care (Davis, McGadney, Barrasi, & Stull, 1993) and were required to rely on internal resources.

Each cultural population has a cultural history and tradition that is unique and different. There is often a tendency to describe different cultural groups as being homogeneous. To do so limits the potential for designing and implementing programs that are cost-efficient and effective. Responding to groups in stereotypic fashion interferes and hinders attempts to effective intervention. Diversity within each population may actually be greater than that between the various ethnic groups. This is a vital distinction that is essential to fully understand ethnic individuals, families, and their behavior.

At the risk of overgeneralizing, there are some broad differences that are inherent to all ethnic groups in contrast to western European American values. These differences are crucial in deciphering and describing cultural/ethnic groups and, ultimately, in being able to provide the supports needed to enhance the caregiving process. A first difference is that ethnic groups seem to have a more collectivistic orientation as opposed to the individualistic orientation of white American families (Laungani & Palmer, 2002). The social structure and decision-making perspective of a collectivistic orientation goes beyond the individual. Rather than taking the perspective that only the individual makes and benefits from a decision, the collectivistic perspective considers how decisions affect the entire family, often even beyond the immediate family. Issues are explored from a broader perspective than from just that of the individual.

This collectivistic type of decision-making is taken for granted in most Asian and Hispanic cultures, but an important corollary to this perspective is the reliance of the individual on the extended family. This is a significant departure from the individualistic or independent view that is characteristic of American society, and has implications for service provision. Following a series of focus groups with eight ethnic-specific populations, Scharlach and colleagues (2006) concluded that programs and services that met needs of individual caregivers rather than the whole family were underutilized by nonwhite caregivers. Despite this finding, an idealized or romanticized perspective of ethnic families should not dominate, and the needs of individuals should not be overlooked (Aranda & Knight, 1997; Rosenthal, 1986).

A second major difference between ethnic populations and the white middle class orientation is that ethnic groups generally approach life with a more fatalistic viewpoint. Fatalism can be viewed as a continuum. The general American orientation is to attempt to control the environment rather than merely accepting fate. This perspective is typified by the medical approach of western medicine to cure disease and treat disability in a similar manner. The focus is on treating illness "as an episodic, intrapersonal deviation" that is "person-centered, temporally bounded and discontinuous" (Landrine & Klonoff, 1992, p. 268). Ethnic groups such as African Americans or Hispanic Americans are more likely than white middle class Americans to perceive disabling conditions as a natural part of life. Landrine and Klonoff (1992) described how many ethnic groups viewed the treatment of disease "as a long term, informal, highly personal and cooperative process" (p. 268). Some Hispanic families may view having a child with a disability as an honor that has been bestowed on them because they have the strength to handle such a child.

A third major difference between ethnic groups and mainstream middle class America is particularly relevant to caregiving, namely the issue of independence. Independence is often seen as the primary objective of the rehabilitation process and has become a primary aspiration for people with disabilities. American culture, following from the notion of individualism, places great value on an individual being independent and self-sufficient. Within the brain injury context, independent living has become a permanent part of the rehabilitation lexicon. However, the notion of independent living can be confusing to people from cultures that do not value independence as a primary objective or goal.

Socioeconomic Status

Other aspects such as socioeconomic status further confound much of what is known about ethnic groups and disabilities. Many individuals and families in ethnic groups have lower incomes and fewer resources than white Americans. Indeed, some researchers have suggested that socioeconomic status may be a better predictor of filial support than cultural background (Rosenthal, 1986). Because poverty rates are higher for these groups compared with whites (U.S. Census Bureau, 2011), inability to purchase formal support can result greater reliance only on family. Individuals who cannot afford external resources may be forced to provide care, but this may not necessarily be because of a cultural belief or expectation. The relationship between socioeconomic status, disability, ethnicity, and caregiving remains unknown, but in need of further research. Simply looking at people in terms of their economic status to the exclusion of their cultural dimensions can detract from understanding what is important (Valle, 1998). Whether caregiving is predicated on ethnicity or on socioeconomic status is currently speculative (Tennstedt & Chang, 1998).

Perception of Need

Kosloski, Montgomery, and Karner (1999), in a review of the role of cultural factors in caregiving, indicated that caregivers from ethnic groups "cannot be expected to view their caregiving responsibilities in the same way [as white Americans] because cultural and background differences are likely to moderate perceptions of need" (p. 40). Ethnic differences have been found to influence expectations of assistance as well as the perception of whether caregiving is perceived as strain or burden (Mui, Choi, & Monk, 1998). For instance, among some American Indian groups, people who vary either physically or intellectually are afforded "slightly greater leeway in their behavior" based on recognition that disability is beyond an individual or family's control (Pengra & Godfrey, 2001). Pengra and Godfrey (2001) elaborated on how disability is simply accepted in some ethnic cultures as a part of life, and therefore something to be managed along with many other things. These beliefs may lead to a tendency to overlook the need for formal services (Aranda & Knight, 1997). Marks (1995) found that in the greater New Orleans area that African American caregivers indicated the lowest level of perceived burden and white caregivers indicated the highest level. The cognitive status of the care receiver was not significantly associated with perceived level of burden (Marks, 1995; Mui et al., 1998). Among American Indian families, Pengra and Godfrey (2001) noted that people with disabilities often received assistance as part of a family's normal routine. "Kinship responsibilities are an indivisible and un-defined force" (Pengra & Godfrey, 2001, p. 39) and as such caregiving was not considered to be help. Further, Pengra and Godfrey (2001) suggested that receiving assistance from family members did not make the recipient feel powerless or pitied, but rather a loved and a fully functioning member of the family.

Davis and colleagues (1993) described the role that perceived cause of illness might play in caregiving, citing a 74-year-old female who said, "I can put up with the pain because arthritis runs in the family and all of us get it when we reach our fifties" (p. 78). She chose to live without assistance knowing that her situation was considered to be normal and what was expected in her family. Understanding the perception or view of a disabling condition and its etiology, and the interaction between this and the cultural and/or traditional roles of family and family members is critical to understanding the caregiving process within ethnic groups. For instance, viewing brain injury as the result of punishment or sanction for personal behavior is common in many ethnic populations (Landrine & Klonoff, 1992). Although these beliefs are not unique to ethnic populations (Landrine & Klonoff, 1992), the belief that disability results from the behavior of the individual or a family member may dictate the caregiving response of the family. Guilt associated with the belief that the injury results from sanctions for misbehavior may reinforce the notion that caregiving is an obligation and even a necessary atonement for previous transgressions.

Indeed, a sense of obligation is often found in Asian American families and is a motivating force for caregiving. This is especially the case in Chinese culture where there is an expectation that one's children will be the source of long-term care for the elderly. Yu, Kim, Liu, and Wong (1993) suggested that cultural belief goes beyond issues of affordability or economics but focusses on what should be even when this aspiration cannot be met in reality.

Conclusion
The task of caregiving for people with brain injuries in ethnic populations is not that different from the more traditional mainstream groups.

However, much is lacking in our knowledge of how ethnicity and culture impact on the caregiving process with people who have disabilities. Little is known about the practice of caregiving across cultures and different ethnic groups. Although lip service is often given to the need to attend to ethnicity and culture in current policy, there are no specific policies that focus on this topic. Worse, policies assume that what is good for one group will be sufficient for another. A more tailored approach to caregiving is required that is flexible and open to both individual and cultural variations. Services that achieve this will undoubtedly be more effective and acceptable to different cultural groups. All citizens with brain injuries and their families deserve the best support possible, regardless of their ethnicity. The National Institute on Minority Health and Health Disparities (2012) suggests that culturally competent methods and interventions to support caregiving need to become standard components of any health delivery system. Although the practice of caregiving within ethnic populations result in the same needs as in any population, because people who are from ethnic groups are more likely to have fewer resources available to them, there is need for service providers to understand factors beyond those that affect the white middle class. Further, the motivations of ethnic families for providing care may be different to those found in more westernized middle class families. Different ethnic groups may perceive the process of caregiving in ways that may not make sense to observers from outside those groups. Service providers seeking to engage families from diverse populations who are dealing with brain injury need to appreciate these perspectives in designing and implementing support programs. There is also a need for programs to understand the diversity within various ethnic groups and where particular individuals or families stand with regard to their acceptance and adoption of American values (Valle, 1998).

Ethnic groups exist within a host society that influences their values and interactions. Thus they continue to evolve following their initial migration and where any particular family may be on the acculturation continuum has implications for their caregiving or lack of caregiving behavior. An awareness and understanding of the multidimensionality of acculturation (Aranda & Knight, 1997) can go a long ways toward assisting these ethnic populations to utilize available community supports that enhance their own ability to provide care to persons with disabilities.

Because of the growing population of people who have disabilities resulting from brain injury, there will be a need for "new solutions that affect the social structure and function of society" (Hooyman & Gonyea, 1995, p. 263). Hooeyman and Gonyea (1995) elaborated that the underlying conflicting values of individualism, familism, and societal good will continue to need attention. Similarly Gelfand and Yee (1991) emphasized the importance of addressing language and acculturation in service provision. Acknowledgement of the impact of ethnicity and culture on the caregiving process can open up the potential for ethnic families with disabilities to bring to knowledge and dialogue about caregiving that could inform the next generation. It is likely that ethnic populations have much to teach us about the ways of caregiving, irrespective of cultural differences.

Acknowledgment

I wish to acknowledge the assistance of Kelly Leinweber in the preparation of this chapter.

References

American Association of Retired Persons (AARP) (2001). *In the middle: a report on multicultural boomers coping with family and aging issues. A national survey*. Retrieved from AARP website: http://research.aarp.org/il/inthemiddle1.html

American Association of Retired Persons (AARP) (2004). *Caregiving in the United States*. Retrieved from http://www.caregiving.org/data/04finalreport.pdf

American Association of Retired Persons (AARP) (2009). *Caregiving in the U.S. 2009*. Retrieved from http://www.caregiving.org/data/Caregiving_in_the_US_2009_full_report.pdf

Angel, R., & Tienda, M. (1982). Determinants of extended household structure: Cultural pattern or economic need? *American Journal of Sociology, 87*(6), 1360–1383.

Aranda, M. P., & Knight, B. G. (1997). The influence of ethnicity and culture on the caregiver stress and coping process: a sociocultural review and analysis. *The Gerontologist, 37*(3), 342–354.

Bethell, C., & Lansky, D., & Fiorillo, J. (2001). *A portrait of the chronically ill in America, 2001*. Princeton, NJ: Robert Wood Johnson Foundation.

Cantor, M. H., Gelfand, D. E., & Kutzik, A (1979). The informal support system of New York's inner city elderly: Is ethnicity a factor? In D. E. Gelfand, & A. J. Kutzik. (Eds.), *Ethnicity and aging: Theory, research and policy*. New York: Springer.

Collins, K. S., Hughes, D. L., Doty, M. M., Ives, B. L., Edwards, J. N., & Tenney, K. (2002). *Diverse communities, common concerns: Assessing health care quality for minority Americans*. Retrieved from The Commonwealth Fund: http://www.commonwealthfund.org/~/media/Files/Publications/Fund%20Report/2002/Mar/Diverse%20Communities%20%20Common%20Concerns%20%20Assessing%20Health%20Care%20Quality%20for%20Minority%20Americans/collins_diversecommun_523%20pdf.pdf

Cox, C., Monk, A., Barresi, C. M., & Stull, D. E. (1993). *Black and Hispanic caregivers of dementia victims in ethnic elderly and long term care*. New York: Springer.

Davis, L. H., McGadney, B. F., Barrasi, C. M., & Stull, D. E. (1993). *Self-care practices of black elders in ethnic elderly and long term care*. New York: Springer.

Feinberg, L. F., Gray, L., & Kelly, K. A. (2002). *Family caregiving as a grantmaking area: Current focus and future trends*. San Francisco, CA: Family Caregiver Alliance.

Gelfand, D., & Yee, B. Y. K. (1991). Trends and forces: Influence of immigration, migration and acculturation on the fabric of aging in America. *Generations, 15*(4), 7–10.

Hooyman, N. R., & Gonyea, J. (1995). *Feminist perspectives on family care*. Thousand Oaks, CA: Sage.

Kosloski, K., Montgomery, R. J., & Karner, T. X. (1999). Differences in the perceived need for assistive services by culturally diverse caregivers of persons with dementia. *Journal of Applied Gerontology, 18*(2), 239–256.

Landrine, H., & Klonoff, E. A. (1992). Culture and health-related schemas: A review and proposal for interdisciplinary integration. *Health Psychology, 11*(4), 267–276.

Laungani, P., & Palmer, S. (2002). *Understanding mental illness across cultures in multicultural counseling.* London: Sage.

Lefley, H. P. (1996). *Family caregiving in mental illness.* Thousand Oaks, CA: Sage.

Lubben, J. E., Becerra, R. M., Gelfand, D. E., & Barressi, C. M. (1987). *Social support among Black, Mexican, and Chinese elderly in research and ethnic dimensions of aging.* New York: Springer.

Mui, A. C., Choi, N. G., & Monk, A. (1998). *Long-term care and ethnicity.* Westport, CT: Auburn House.

National Council on Disability. (1993). *Meeting the unique needs of minorities with disabilities: a report to the President and the Congress.* Retrieved from http://www.eric.ed.gov/PDFS/ED357526.pdf

National Institute on Minority Health and Health Disparities. (2012). Retrieved from http://www.nimhd.nih.gov/about_ncmhd/mission.asp

Navaie-Waliser, M., Feldman, P. H., Gould, D. A., Levine, C., Kuerbis, A. N., & Donelan, K. (2001). The experiences and challenges of informal caregivers: common themes and differences among whites, blacks, and hispanics. *The Gerontologist, 41*(6), 733–741.

Ory, M. G., Hoffman, R. R., Yee, J., Tennstedt, S., & Schultz, R. (1999). Prevalence and impact of caregiving: a detailed comparison. *The Gerontologist, 39*(2), 177–185.

Pask, E. G. (2000). Culture: caring and curing in the changing health scene. In: J. D. Morgan (Ed.). *Meeting the needs of our clients creatively: Impact of art and culture on caregiving.* Amityville, NY: Baywood Publishing Co.

Pengra, L. M., & Godfrey, J. G. (2001). Different boundaries, different barriers: Disability studies and Lakota Culture. *Disability Studies Quarterly, 21*(3), 36–53.

Rosenthal, C. J. (1986). Family supports in later life: Does ethnicity makes a difference? *The Gerontologist, 26*(1), 19–24.

Scharlach, A. E., Kellam, R., Ong, N., Baskin, A., Goldstein, C., & Fox, P. J. (2006). Cultural attitudes and caregiver service use: lessons from focus groups with racially and ethnically diverse family caregivers. *Journal of Gerontological Social Work, 47*(1–2), 133–156.

Smart, J., & Smart, D. W. (1997). The racial/ethnic demography of disability. *Journal of Rehabilitation, 63*(4), 9–15.

Sue, D. W., & Sue, D. (2002). *Counseling the culturally diverse* (4th ed.). New York: Wiley.

Tennstedt, S., & Chang, B. (1998). The relative contribution of ethnicity versus socioeconomic status in explaining differences in disability and receipt of informal care. *The Journal of Gerontology, 53*(2), 561–570.

U.S. Census Bureau. (2011). Income, Poverty and Health Insurance Coverage in the U.S. Retrieved from census.gov/prud/2011pubs/60–239.pdf

U.S. Department of Health and Human Services. (2002). *Self-evaluation to promote community living for people with disabilities.* Retrieved from http://www.hhs.gov/newfreedom/final/hhsappenda.html

U.S. Surgeon General, U.S. Department of Health and Human Services. (2002). *Mental health: Culture, race and ethnicity.* Rockville, MD: Author.

Valle, R. (1998). *Caregiving across cultures.* New York: Taylor & Francis.

Wagner, D. L. (1997) *Comparative analysis of caregiver data for caregivers to the elderly, 1987–1997,* National Alliance for Caregiving, Bethesda, MD. Retrieved from immn.org/pdf/research/analysis/pdf

Wood, J. B., & Wan, T. T. H. (1992). Ethnicity and minority issues in family caregiving to rural black elders. In M. C. Barresi, & E. D. Stull (Eds.). *Ethnicity and long-term care.* New York: Springer.

World Health Organization (WHO) (2000). *International classification of functioning, disability, and health.* Available from: http://www.who.int/classifications/icf/en/

Young, R. F., & Kahana, E. (1995). The context of caregiving and well-being outcomes among African and Caucasian Americans. *The Gerontologist, 35*(2), 225–232.

Yu, E. S., Kim, H., Liu, W. T., & Wong, S. (1993). Functional abilities of Chinese and Korean elders in congregate housing. In C. M. Barresi & D. E. Stull (Eds.). *Ethnic elderly and long term care.* New York: Springer.

CHAPTER 15

Community Leaders within a Brain Injury Self-management Program: A Valuable Resource

Heidi Muenchberger, Areti Kennedy, and Elizabeth Kendall

Engaging with the Community

The community setting is the best context from which to support people with traumatic brain injury (TBI) in the long term (Winkler, Unsworth, & Sloan, 2006). Given that individuals with brain injury experience difficulties re-integrating into the community following hospital-based rehabilitation, facilitating stronger networks within local communities is a key step in establishing positive and sustainable outcomes for individuals and their families. In brain injury rehabilitation, knowledge of community support networks and health programs delivered by community-based services are significantly underdeveloped, resulting in heightened risk of underutilization of community resources in favor of hospital-based services (Muenchberger, Kendall, & Neal, 2008). In recent years, programs delivered by community members are emerging as an important focus for brain injury rehabilitation support over the longer term. This chapter examines the experiences of community-based program leaders who have delivered a brain injury specific skill-based course aimed at developing and capitalizing on local support networks for people with acquired brain injury (ABI) and their families.

Rehabilitation interventions based within the community have been found to facilitate the social and community integration of individuals with TBI, even many years after injury (Petrella, McColl, Krupa, & Johnston, 2005). However, the ability of individuals to meaningfully participate as full members in their community in the long term is often limited by the dearth of opportunities and the lack of appropriate supports to facilitate this natural social interaction. Returning to the community after TBI is challenging, not least because of the lack of structured community support available. Education and general support groups often fail due to lack of a formal engagement process, lack of supervision and planning, and lack of sustainability measures. One way of better supporting people with injuries and developing community involvement is through networks of peer support that offer a structured approach to learning and participation (Barlow, Bancroft, & Turner, 2004; Kennedy, Rogers, & Gately, 2005).

Community leaders can be defined as lay people (i.e., peer leaders) as well as health professionals (i.e., health professional leaders) who are based within the community. They usually undergo an intensive period of training by a host organization to deliver a specific educational program to a client group. Given that leaders are potentially people who have experienced injury themselves, the engagement of peer leaders is a particularly powerful intervention strategy in itself. Peer learning models are based on the principles of social learning theory, which identifies role modeling as an important component of the learning process (Turner & Shepherd, 1999). These models have become popular in health promotion in recent years, based on the belief that peer influence may be more credible and more readily accepted than that of health professional experts.

In the brain injury field, recent focus of these programs has been twofold: (1) a psychoeducational component aimed at increasing personal knowledge of injury and its management and (2) a social component emphasizing collective goal formation and enactment to build support networks. Despite the growing acceptance of the efficacy of such peer support programs, there is limited knowledge about the experiences and perceptions of the community leaders themselves and how systems and communities can facilitate and support such networks.

One program that promotes the involvement of peer leaders is the STEPS (Skills to Enable People and Communities) program, an educationally based support program managed by the Acquired Brain Injury Outreach Service (ABIOS) in Queensland, Australia.

The STEPS program which has operated since 2005 aims to improve the psychosocial, health, and environmental outcomes for people with traumatic and acquired brain injury and their families by enhancing community participation and creating networks of support in local communities. The networks of supports are developed through the implementation of an educational program (i.e., the STEPSSkills Program), which is delivered by a local community facilitator or leader. The main purpose of the STEPS program is to share knowledge about brain injury and learn from others' experiences while forming connections with the local community.

Overview of the STEPS Program

The STEPS Program consists of the following phases: (1) The STEPS Skills Program; and (2) The STEPS Network Groups.

(1) The STEPS Skills Program comprises six, weekly sessions delivered in a small group format, each session lasting two hours in duration. The content and structure of the STEPS course is outlined in Table 15.1. The course provides education and strategies to individuals with brain injury and their families about how to self-manage with injury ("How I look after myself"), how to engage in the community ("How I live in the community"), and how to work with community services. An integral and final component of the course comprises a planned group activity, which is intended to provide participants with an opportunity to experience a positive social outing together. This group activity aims to develop participant skills in planning and carrying out their own community activity.

(2) The STEPS Network Groups are typically formed by participants who have completed the STEPS Skills Program, offering the opportunity for them to maintain the connections they have developed during the initial six-week program. The structure of STEPS network groups differs according to the needs and preferences of specific groups, though most groups continue to meet on a monthly rather than weekly basis.

Leader Recruitment and Training

Community-based leaders are recruited through an active engagement strategy by ABIOS working with local communities to gauge local capacity and interest in STEPS Program delivery in multiple locations around Queensland, Australia. All potential leaders are provided with a role description, code of conduct, volunteer agreement, and leader application form (requiring referees and professional details). Following this formal application process, ABIOS determines the suitability of leaders for the program, establishes contact with these leaders, and registers them on a leader database.

Program leaders are members of the local community who have either experienced a brain injury themselves, or are a family member/friend of a person with a brain injury, collectively termed "peer leaders," or could otherwise be health or disability professionals. All leaders engage in the program on a voluntary basis, although a reimbursement package for travel expenses is available to eligible leaders. A key component of the STEPS program is the purposeful establishment of local peer-professional partnerships for program delivery, i.e. a peer leader co-leading with a health or disability professional.

Each session is guided by a STEPS Program workbook to ensure consistency of the course information and activities. Each participant is

229

Table 15.1 STEPS course content

Session		Content
Session 1	Introduction To Program	About Self-Management
Session 2	How I Look After Myself	Goal setting Understanding acquired brain injury Changes after brain injury
Session 3	How I Look After Myself	Managing stress Working on specific problems after brain injury
Session 4	How I Look After Myself	Getting structure and balance in my life
	How I Live In The Community	Relationships with family and friends Relationships with other people Linking with friends
Session 5	How I Live In The Community How I Work With Services	Common difficulties in the community Exploring activities and experiences Our group future Risk taking How I work with services
Session 6	Our Group Break Up Activity	

provided with a workbook divided into each of the session topic areas. Throughout the course, participants are encouraged to reflect on their own experiences, and share their ideas and stories with the group. Leaders are provided with a Leader workbook, which contains additional group facilitation notes and training tips. A final break up activity in Session 6 is intended to capitalize on the social interactions formed within the group as well as the skills gained in planning and goal setting. Program content also specifically addresses group members' interest in continuing to meet and support each other beyond the duration of the STEPS Skills Program, using the skills and processes learned in the course to develop a sustainable social network, or STEPS Network group.

In a study conducted by Griffith University, Australia, 18 community-based leaders volunteered to share their experiences of the program. The majority of the leaders were female (78%) and half of the eight peer leaders were over the age of 55 years. Five of the peer leaders had experienced a brain injury (traumatic brain injury, $n = 3$; stroke, $n = 2$) themselves, while the remaining three peer leaders were family members of people who had experienced a brain injury ($n = 2$) or a spouse ($n = 1$). None of the peer leaders were currently in full-time paid work, and the majority

(75%) had undertaken some form of volunteer work prior to their commencement of the leader training course. Previous occupations held by peer leaders included a nurse, teacher, fire-fighter, human resource manager, crane driver, waiter, and interior decorator.

Most (60%, $n = 6$) of the ten health professional leaders in the sample had delivered their first course within 3 months of completing training. On average, health professionals delivered their first course almost two months after completion of leader training. For peer leaders, the average

Table 15.2 Demographic details of the leader sample at review

Demographics	Health Professional Leaders (n=10)	Peer Leaders (n=8)	Overall % (n=18)
Gender (female)	90%	63%	78 (14)
Age (av):			
20–30	67%	13%	36 (5)
31–50	17%	37%	28 (4)
55+	17%	50%	36 (5)
With acquired brain injury	10%	62%	33 (6)
Marital status:			
Never married	40%	13%	28 (5)
Married or de facto	40%	36%	50 (9)
Divorced, separated, or widowed	20%	25%	22 (4)
Education:			
High school	10%	26%	17 (3)
Apprenticeship, certificate, or diploma	—	63%	28 (5)
Completed university	90%	13%	56 (10)
Employment status:			
Full-time paid work	60%	—	33 (6)
Volunteer work	—	88%	39 (7)
Part-time paid work	30%	13%	22 (4)
Not in labor force	10%	—	6 (1)

Note: All participants in this review were from English-speaking background and no Culturally and Linguistically Diverse (CALD) participants were identified.

time between training completion and course delivery was 4.3 months. The evident time lag between training and course delivery was dependent on the referral of sufficient course participants in order to justify the delivery of the course in the local area.

Key themes relating to the experience of being a program leader (either peer or health professional leader), course delivery, and future training opportunities are discussed below.

On Becoming a Community Leader

Core motivations for undertaking the role of a STEPS Program leader included the need for a sense of social justice and reciprocity, and the opportunity for self-development.

Social Justice and Reciprocity. Issues of social justice and reciprocity were clearly identified as key motivators for participation in leader training, presumably because of their personal identification with brain injury. They were inspired by the satisfaction they gained from helping others; the desire to reduce the social isolation experienced by people with brain injury; and the desire to provide social justice and equity in service delivery for people with disability.

Peer leaders identified this program as an opportunity to give something back to society after having experienced their own injury and rehabilitation. Volunteering as a leader was seen as a way of facilitating a more positive process for other effected individuals by sharing their personal experiences: "I have come a long way in my recovery, and I want others to reach the same level" and "I want to share the wonderful post-ABI life with others . . . and give people hope"(Peer Leader).

Another peer leader spoke about the benefits he had gained from previously participating in a course and wanted to impart the sense of social support and belonging that the course had given him throughout his rehabilitation journey:

> I wanted to help other people as I had been helped . . . I felt that I had benefited from attending my first STEPS course and I was hoping that other people would get the same help . . . yeah it opened my eyes . . . I felt alive . . . I felt I wasn't alone anymore . . . it was a wonderful feeling of belonging . . . It was like I was with likeminded people that I had known for a long time. (Peer Leader)

Recognizing a Service Gap. All leaders indicated the desire to provide a new service to an at-risk-and-in-need group within their local community, and expressed their belief in the benefits of this course to individuals with brain injury residing in the community. Specifically, peer leaders identified the lack of local services, appropriate postacute rehabilitation, and brain-injury-specific programs. They viewed the course as a way of overcoming this service gap: "I have a partner who has an acquired brain injury and we have been searching for support groups—we joined the group so we could benefit and the community"; "[We] need something in the local area," "Services are not appropriate for ABI" (Peer Leaders).

Health professionals similarly reported a lack of postacute, community-based rehabilitation options for individuals with ABI and their families, particularly in communities located outside the metropolitan area. Thus, there was a need to remediate the lack of community rehabilitation services for outpatients, as one health professional mentioned, "There is not much follow-up from the hospital into the community and STEPS was a way to do this." As indicated in the peer leader data, health professional leaders were motivated to deliver the STEPS course due to the lack of specialist brain injury rehabilitation services in their community. Health professional leaders confirmed that the STEPS course provided an important and unique community rehabilitation service, particularly in regional areas where community options for rehabilitation were limited or unavailable.

Health professionals reported that structured support groups, such as STEPS, was a way to formally engage people with brain injuries and their families in rehabilitation, "The STEPS course was considered a structured intervention targeted towards a group that I currently work with." They further identified the lack of age-appropriate services for younger people with brain injury, and viewed the STEPS course as an important community service.

> A colleague and myself identified that we were having a lot of clients' come through [another] program with stroke or brain injury . . . we started to identify that these people were a lot younger than our regular clients. We are a service that provides services for aged and people with disabilities . . . mostly people in their seventies access our services, but we had noticed a cluster of much younger people coming through. So I was really at the point of looking for some training around stroke and working with younger people that have experienced brain injury. (Health Professional Leader)

Self-development. All leaders perceived the STEPS Skills Program to be an opportunity to increase their knowledge and develop skills in group facilitation. Self-education was a key motivator for peer leaders who expressed a desire to increase their knowledge about brain injury and its consequences. The course was also seen as a way of acquiring valuable skills in group facilitation: "[being trained as a course leader] would give me a better understanding of the injury and how to deliver the training" (Peer Leader). Some peer leaders were already coordinators of a local stroke or brain injury support group, and wanted to extend their skills

233

through more formal leader training. For some peer leaders, the receipt of training had the potential to assist with gaining competitive employment: "ultimately, [I] want to gain some skills for paid employment" (Peer Leader).

For many, the positive nature of their previous volunteering experiences was a motivating factor in joining in the STEPS Program leader-training course. One peer leader described how her previous experience as a volunteer was an important training ground that had nurtured her desire to impart the message of acceptance and hope for people with disabilities:

> I was an event director for dressage [horse riding] . . . I loved it . . . I didn't get involved in competing, but I had a buzz. I was amazed when people would come up to speak to me and then within seconds they accepted me in my wheelchair . . . that's what I wanted to get across to people, sure, I have a disability, but I am a person. (Peer Leader)

Knowledge Development: Increasing Specialist Skills and Understanding of Brain Injury. As was the case with peer leaders, health professional leaders viewed the leader course and subsequent delivery of the STEPS course as a unique opportunity to augment their current knowledge base and gain specific skills in managing brain injury. Working directly with people with brain injury through the STEPS course also satisfied their need as health professionals to support the brain injury population and enhance an individual's quality of life by providing much needed education and a community service, for example, "I have worked closely with ABI patients over a twelve year period and am interested in supporting their long term quality of life and any ongoing issues" (Health Professional Leader). Peer leaders considered the course topics to be slightly more relevant and useful to them compared to some health professional leaders. This finding may reflect the fact that peer leaders had, for the first time, gained important knowledge about brain injury and were able to relate their personal experiences to a knowledge base.

Leader Experiences of the Course Delivery

Overall, the leaders viewed the course as influential, particularly in relation to its objective of expanding social support networks. Their experiences of the course delivery process highlighted both success factors and potential barriers to the sustainability of the program. These factors mainly included the context of co-facilitation, group cohesion; course structure, and organizational support.

The Benefits of Co-facilitation. Co-facilitation was identified as a useful strategy to enhance client learning and facilitate leader workloads. Peer leaders recognized the benefits of sharing the workload between two people (where one person has a brain injury), "co-facilitation is the main reason why I decided to go ahead with the course delivery, I knew [the health professional leader] would help me if I needed it, it was wonderful having the [health professional leader] and her experience" (Peer Leader).

Co-facilitation also provided peer leaders with an opportunity to share their valuable personal experience with the support of their co-leader. Indeed, peer leaders indicated that the STEPS course was a source of validation of their ability to deliver an education service to their community and to be recognized appropriately for this, "It was nice to be taken seriously, it made you feel worthwhile" and "I would like to try and do it on my own, but given my difficulties in my personal life, there is no way I would have done it on my own . . . sometimes what one will pick up the other one will, so it is good to co-facilitate, sometimes if both have brain injury, you don't pick up things like you would have before"(Peer Leader).

Co-facilitation for health professional leaders also meant sharing workloads and promoting the STEPS message, "I was very keen to promote the STEPS group and the STEPS program within my team . . . as it's a kind of new area for us . . . and I was keen to get on board my team members' interest and they were very responsive to the idea of STEPS." Health professionals highlighted the different styles evident between peer leaders and health professionals, and the need to discuss and clarify approaches, "with one [leader] wanting to follow the program and the other wanting to be a lot looser with the program structure . . ." Another health professional was happy to co-facilitate in the short term, and perceived her role as an ancillary one that aimed to develop skills within the peer leader and provide support for them to deliver the course independently in future.

> My interest is in motivating clients and stroke support groups — ABI support groups were saying they wouldn't mind someone with a professional background as a support person that could run their first groups. Then once they felt confident I would back off and let them run with it. (Health Professional Leader)

Group Cohesion: Meaningful Interaction Beyond the Course Context. Peer leaders highlighted the social nature of the course and the benefits of this for facilitating meaningful interaction beyond the course context. However, for some leaders, the need for social interaction sometimes came at the expense of progressing the course content, as one peer leader explained: "some of them [course participants] live on their own, they love company and love to keep talking, and you have to try and say, 'we'll stick to this for the moment,' and we usually say for half an hour we can talk later . . ." (Peer Leader).

As group cohesion developed, so did the commitment to the group. For example, one leader described how the group responded to a crisis involving one of its members, engendering a feeling of support and belonging: "One person had three [seizures] one night and broke his leg and was hospitalized, and at the end of the course one of the ABI carers was taken ill and had to leave the group . . . but we visited them, gave them a lot of support, they felt so much a part of the group"(Peer Leader). One peer leader referred to the term family when reflecting on his experiences of group cohesion, due to the genuine nature of the interactions and trust in each other's experience.

Building respect amongst group participants was identified as being integral to group cohesion as mutual respect encouraged sharing and meaningful feedback: "You have to have a lot of respect for the group and then you can ask respect from them . . . that way they open up to you, building trust within the group and the feedback becomes real" (Peer Leader). It was observed that the small group-training format facilitated this sharing process, particularly as it provided an opportunity to listen to questions from others and learn together. This established a culture of shared learning and social support that continued into ongoing STEPS Network Groups.

> The group decided to meet once a month, and alternately one month will be a formal get together where the group members only would attend, and the next month informal, family and friends will also attend and we would go out to a picnic. (Peer Leader)

Some peer leaders reported that they met after the final social event to catch up with each other and have made plans for ongoing contact, thus suggesting an unintended positive outcome of expanded social networks for the leaders themselves, not just the group participants.

Given that the purpose of the STEPS Skills Program was to facilitate sustainable social support networks through enhanced community participation, the role of leaders as integral members of this network was critical. Peer leaders searched for ways of facilitating greater interaction and social engagement amongst participants. Despite this commitment to social engagement, peer leaders noted that not all participants engaged in social events.

Benefits of a Structured Course with Organizational Support. All leaders described the benefits of working with a structured (i.e., program-based) course: "Having a script and structure to work by was important [although] keeping the groups on time was a major challenge." Some leaders adjusted the structure to suit their own style and preferred delivery mode, using the workbook as a general guide rather than following the suggested structure rigidly. This meant that they could pursue further discussion on topics as the need arose. Other leaders found that adherence to the structure enabled them to keep the group more focused on the activities for that particular session. Regardless of the method leaders used, they all appreciated the structure that was provided.

Leaders stated that the support received from the host organization was essential. Administrative support (i.e., providing workbooks, locating potential clients, finding venues, checking in, responding to need, and providing supervision and ongoing support) was similarly regarded as an important facilitator of successful courses: "I had access to all the resources I needed. All the participant workbooks were prepared for me, and [this support] allowed me to run the course" (Peer Leader).

The training and preparation of peer leaders was complementary to their personal situation, which was highly valued.

For instance, peer leaders expressed gratitude that the organization supported them in their own personal difficulties: "I thought [the support from the organization] was wonderful . . . they gave me support in my personal life, I'm so grateful, I needed help and support to enable me to continue [with the program]"(Peer Leader). For health professionals, the opportunity to pre-plan and then debrief with ABIOS, especially in regard to session planning, was extremely useful, "I had the opportunity to debrief with ABIOS after every session and also talk to them before every session just to make sure I was clear on what I wanted to present and that I did in fact have all the information" (Health Professional Leader).

Future Training Opportunities for Community Leaders

Information about the Brain, Disability, and the Adjustment Process. One area of particular training need identified by peer leaders who did not have any first-hand experience of brain injury was the physical manifestations of brain injury, i.e., the neurological focus of ABI and "anything to do with the brain."

There was also interest in learning more about the impact of disability on individuals and families. For instance, peer leaders mentioned that some group participants were still dealing with the impact and trauma of the brain injury. In this case, the peer leader explained that "some hold grudges; they transfer the blame of the accident [to other people]." Peer leaders wanted to understand more about the natural course of brain injury and the adjustment process, "the brain injury trajectory," particularly in relation to the needs of older people with brain injury who have had difficulties coping with their disability, "[my brother-in-law] is 62 and in a wheelchair [and doesn't do much for himself], is this his way of coping? I don't know."

The issue of establishing leader–participant boundaries and clear role identification was articulated by peer leaders, and was particularly pertinent in small communities. Peer leaders were cognizant of breeching privacy of program participants during group processes and information sharing "[at the first meeting] I was worried that I might invade their privacy . . . it's a big issue these days . . . I had to read up and had training"; "I already knew half the group . . . I felt 80% at ease but a little bit concerned about everyone's privacy" (Peer Leader). Given that the STEPS Skills Program focuses on establishing a circle of friends and a social support network, important questions were raised about the extent to which the leader can be involved in this circle of friends.

Attending to the needs of individuals who have stabilized in their injury course, and understanding adjustment and imparting strategies to assist was clearly important for peer leaders who were carers for their aging friend or relative.

Opportunities for In-depth Learning. In relation to the process of learning, peer leaders identified that additional courses and case scenarios were potentially useful approaches in facilitating their learning. For instance, advanced leader training was suggested as a method to gain a deeper appreciation of some of the issues mentioned in the course, "an optional advanced course might be a useful strategy for further training—as a follow up course." For example, peer leaders expressed interest in information and skills in how to deal with the injury-related behavioral difficulties that may arise within the group context. One peer leader suggested, "training on how to deal with this [brain injury] in the context of the course, and having some basic counseling skills to diffuse a situation." Another peer leader considered that presenting case scenarios about brain injury, and subsequent challenges faced by individuals with brain injury (e.g., cognitive, behavioral, emotional, social) would provide additional guidance to peer leaders who had no direct experience with brain injury, and allow them to enhance their STEPS course delivery by considering individual needs.

However, peer leaders commented that they required more time to become familiar with the training material. Due to the intense nature of the resources and lack of familiarity with concepts/terms, some peer leaders preferred to extend the training out over a number of days rather than the two days currently being offered. In contrast, health professionals wanted a course that consumed less time, given their pressed time schedules and demanding workloads. They suggested that a more intensive course structure would be more suitable (i.e., one full day workshop).

Attending to the Process of Learning. In response to the question of further training needs, health professionals commented on the need to review the processes of leader training, rather than focus on additional brain injury content. A suggestion was made that mini presentations throughout the leader training would be beneficial in reducing any unease regarding the delivery of presentations. In addition, another health professional leader highlighted the need to "focus on positive self evaluation, rather than critical evaluation," thereby considering the leader training as an opportunity for constructive feedback about group process as well as reflecting on the delivery of the course content.

Reinforcing Learning: Refresher Courses. Although not so much an advanced course, health professionals considered that a refresher course might be useful to "keep you familiar with the whole course content." Given the paucity of similar community oriented programs specifically geared toward brain injury, particularly in regional areas, and the time-lag experienced between training and delivering the course in some cases, it was suggested to re-run courses over time to aid as a refresher tool. Many health professionals believed that this would serve to continue the momentum of the STEPS philosophy and reinforce previous learning. Health professionals also believed that on-the-job training was likely to occur in the course of the STEPS delivery, suggesting that with more experience in conducting a course, leaders will be able to learn from clients, and address more focused and meaningful questions that were not necessarily dealt with in the initial training. Other general statements regarding the leader training process from health professionals included information about:

* involving family members as co-participants to aid the clients' understanding of the issues and the processes with which to achieve this
* capitalizing on the experience and guidance from people who have delivered the course in the past
* increasing training in targeted areas of brain injury such as challenging behaviors, understanding the impact of co-morbid conditions such as depression and brain injury, and complex conditions such as psychosis in brain injury.

Discussion

Community leaders are increasingly recognized as an important rehabilitation resource in facilitating self-confidence and social competence following injury or chronic illness. Indeed, they have become an important part of the overall health infrastructure, yet their capacity and commitment for long-term involvement is not well understood. Social support has been described as an unintended or peripheral benefit of community-based education courses. However, the primary rationale as described in the STEPS Skills Program is to develop a local support network, and the skills required to mobilize that network when needed. Thus, the peer leader becomes central in establishing this local social connectivity. Findings from other peer leader studies have shown that leaders experience difficulty balancing time demands of delivering the components of the course in the time frame provided, whilst attending to client questions and facilitating meaningful group discussion (Catalano, Kendall, Vandenberg, & Hunter, 2008). These studies have reported that leaders would benefit from greater host organization support in managing such issues, which may in turn have a positive impact on the sustainability of the group. The increasingly integrated, but potentially isolated, role of leaders presents unique challenges that require further insight and understanding if this model of delivery is to continue to be expanded.

In relation to their motivation to become a program leader, leaders were inspired by altruistic reasons generally, but also by the opportunity to remedy the apparent service gap for people with TBI. Indeed, some leaders believed it was their responsibility as a community member with first-hand knowledge of brain injury to respond in any way possible. Becoming a trained leader was also viewed as a potential stepping-stone to competitive employment, which shifts the focus from volunteerism to the professionalization of a support workforce.

Although there was strong satisfaction with the support provided (training, materials, venue sourcing by the host agency), the leaders highlighted the importance of on-the-ground support within their local communities particularly in areas of boundary setting, role identification, and managing time/resource demands. It was clear that operational support is required for the long-term sustainability of such programs.

This chapter highlights the central and crucial role of community leaders in delivering community-based programs such as the STEPS program. Leaders appeared to have a positive role within the STEPS program and the position can be viewed as a broader partnership between leaders, participants, organizations, and communities.

For similar programs, maximizing leader engagement can be undertaken in three key phases, namely establishment of leaders, involvement of leaders, and maintenance of leaders. Opportunities to enhance leader commitment over the long term are summarized below:

Opportunities to Maximize Leader Engagement

Establishing leaders

Preparation of leaders—Provision of emotional, administrative, and informational support to leaders throughout program (i.e., pre-training, during training, and post-training). Regular contact and follow up, however brief, is important.

Training of leaders—Providing information about adjustment following brain injury raise the possibility of introducing case scenarios and involving past leaders.

Involving leaders

Access to participants—A clear process for liaising with community groups and promote membership.

Understanding *co-facilitation* processes—Consider establishing clear processes for leader co-facilitation—promote peer leaders as knowledgeable experts, and health professionals as learners.

Providing leader *resources*– Continue to provide resources that are high quality and accessible, and encourage leader and participant feedback regarding workbook.

Maintaining leaders

Facilitating leader *partnerships*—Support leader contact and communication with multiple parties (community, participants, and other leaders) and monitor regularly.

Promoting leader *activities*—Identify community-based champions in organizations, and establish a network of supporters to promote the program within the local community.

Facilitating processes of *engagement*—Develop guidelines for clarifying community-based leader roles (health professionals and peer leaders), responsibilities, and boundaries, and incorporating best-practice research.

Creating a supportive *leader network* in future—As discussed in previous research (see Catalano et al., 2007), there is potential for similar programs to establish a statewide leader network or community of support. This requires a formalized and multi-modal system of leader engagement.

While there may be considerable goodwill to take on the role of community leaders in programs aimed to support people with brain injury or other illness, a clear and structured process of engagement, monitoring, and support for leaders remains important and would further strengthen this valuable community role.

References

Barlow, J. H., Bancroft, G. V., & Turner, A. P. (2004). Volunteer, lay tutors' experiences of the chronic disease self-management course: Being valued and adding value. *Health Education Research, 20*(2), 128–136.

Catalano, T., Kendall, E., Vandenberg, A., & Hunter, B. (2008). The experiences of leaders of self-management courses in Queensland: Exploring health professional and peer leaders' perceptions of working together. *Health and Social Care in the Community, 17*(2), 105–115.

Kennedy, A., Rogers, A., & Gately, C. (2005). From patients to providers: Prospects for self-care skills trainers in the National Health Service. *Health and Social Care in the Community, 13*(5), 431–440.

Muenchberger, H., Kendall, E., & Neal, R. (2008). Identity transition following traumatic brain injury: A dynamic process of contraction, expansion and tentative balance. *Brain Injury, 22*(12), 979–992.

Petrella., L., McColl, M. A., Krupa, T., & Johnston, J. (2005). Returning to productive activities: Perspectives of individuals with long-standing acquired brain injuries. *Brain Injury, 19*(9), 643–655.

Turner, G., & Shepherd, J. (1999). A method in search of a theory: Peer education and health promotion. *Health Education Research, 14*(2), 235–247.

Winkler, D., Unsworth, C., & Sloan, S. (2006). Factors that lead to successful community integration following severe traumatic brain injury. *Journal of Head Trauma Rehabilitation, 21*(1), 8–21.

A Last Word: Charting a Positive Course for the Future

Elizabeth Kendall

Each section in this book has raised new possibilities that might not have been thought about a few decades ago. Unfortunately, disability, and especially traumatic brain injury, has been an area steeped in negativity and notions of deficit. The onset of brain injury has rarely been thought of as anything but a personal tragedy, which of course it is in many ways. This negative view of brain injury can be linked to the rise of modern medicine and the biomedical model, which has dominated the way we think about disability. By necessity, medicine has focused on problems that require diagnosis, repair, or cure. Biomedical restorative approaches inherently locate disability as a deficiency within the person, a weakness, or problem that requires expert attention and amelioration. This philosophy has contributed to the marginalization of people with disabilities in society, creating artificial categories that segregate them from their communities. It also gives credence to the false dichotomy between the abled and the disabled.

The social model of disability was based on a strong reaction to the negativity of the biomedical approach. This new approach emphasized the role of broader social factors in determining or contributing to the presence of disability, irrespective of the physical condition of the person. The social model of disability has gained considerable traction over the years, resulting in improved appreciation of people's rights and the need for services that can promote human dignity at all times. There is no doubt that the influence of the social model has been profound, leading to powerful emancipation movements within the disabled community and greater acceptance within the nondisabled community.

However, for some reason, brain injury rehabilitation has been somewhat resistant to the social model. For too long, the focus of the system has remained on problems and losses rather than on positive outcomes or potential. The frustration of many people with brain injury about this focus on negativity has emerged through the stories and experiences contained in this book. Our research over the years has also shown that positive discourses are typically missing in the rehabilitation literature (Sunderland, Catalano, & Kendall, 2009). We found that policy documents and research articles tended to focus on negative terminology with few instances of positive language. In contrast, life story narratives provided by people using their own ways of describing experiences confirmed more instances of humor, positive language, and optimism. This finding suggests that joy and happiness have been discourses that have been silenced in much of the academic and policy debate.

A good example of how negativity can pervade the rehabilitation system lies in the notion of denial, a term which is used regularly in relation to people with brain injuries. Among other things, this term usually refers to the process of setting of goals that appear to exceed the cognitive capacity of the individual. In some circumstances, such goals might be labeled as aspirational, but in the brain injury rehabilitation context, these goals are more likely to be labeled as unachievable and inappropriate. The person may be described as deliberately refusing to accept his or her deficits, lacking in insight or using denial as a pathological form of coping. Although there is some evidence that brain injury may alter one's capacity for accurate self-review, negative labeling by experts is debilitating and places people in a no-win situation, damned for aspiring too high and yet left with no hope and little support to achieve their goals. The defensive denial of deficits may actually be a useful form of coping in the face of severe loss and, indeed, is likely to be used by most of us at some time in our lives. Is it our role in rehabilitation to censor the goals of other people to such an extent? Or is our role simply to facilitate the best possible achievement of those goals within the constraints of each individual's circumstances? How can we refocus our society and our systems so that they acknowledge the seriousness of brain injury, but simultaneously provide the greatest opportunity possible for optimal health and healing?

This book has shown that there are many positive aspects on which to focus our efforts in future. The development of deeper understanding in areas such as neuroplasticity, mindfulness, and resilience has given us positive concepts on which to build better rehabilitation systems and societies for people with brain injuries. These chapters have reminded us about the importance of positive tools, such as playfulness, determination, responsibility, and social support. At a broader level, the chapters in this book have highlighted the importance of positive cultures, collective responses, capacity-building, and health promoting places. The use of these more positive terms does not in any way negate the traumatic loss and grief that is likely to be experienced by those who have suffered brain injury and their families. Instead, this focus simply recognizes that crises are not exclusively negative.

So is it possible that brain injury, although not desirable in any one's life, could be an event that bring benefits? Researchers have begun to document the growth opportunities that may become apparent to us during difficult times, and specifically following traumatic brain injury (McGrath, 2011). In 2012, an article by Professor Stephen Joseph appeared in the London Daily Mail, titled "Trauma can be good for personal growth." The argument underpinning this article is that people often experience growth as a result of the emotional struggle that follows trauma. Although this might be considered an extreme view, our rehabilitation systems could undoubtedly focus more on positive qualities and strengths rather than on deficiencies and problems. Interestingly, there is a growing trend of positivity which has been slowly infiltrating most areas of scholarship, including rehabilitation, over the last decade or so. In the last few years particularly, there has been a literal explosion of articles that adopt a positive stance rather than one based on deficit. Since 2000, the number of publications focusing on positive concepts, such as resilience and flourishing, has quadrupled (Hart & Sasso, 2011). The frequency with which other positive concepts, such as happiness, satisfaction, strengths, and meaning, have been used in the literature has also increased steadily, reinforcing the presence of a positive shift in the dominant way of thinking.

In the rehabilitation sector, this trend has started to translate into recognition that the presence of disability, no matter how severe, does not diminish or eliminate people's strengths and positive qualities (Dunn & Dougherty, 2005). It has allowed us to understand the importance of optimism and hope in the rehabilitation process. It has helped us to see the importance of family and the role family members can play in facilitating recovery. It has encouraged us to develop strengths-based approaches to interventions and to build systems that engage people to become partners in their rehabilitation or designers of their own services. It has taught us to capitalize on the natural positive supports within a person's environment and to appreciate the important role of culture in promoting growth and well-being.

Unfortunately, some critics have misunderstood or misinterpreted the trend toward positivity, likening it in a derogatory way to the popular culture of self-help psychology and labeling it as a Pollyanna-style of thinking, lacking in critical reflection (Kristjansson, 2010). However, rather than being merely the superficial adoption of positive jargon, this trend reflects a deep understanding of the importance of positive qualities in promoting better outcomes for individuals (Naidoo, van den Berg, & Hayes, 2006). At the community level, there has been a similarly resounding shift back to concepts such as civic engagement, public participation, and benevolence in recognition that these movements can bring benefits for many people. Research has begun to acknowledge the role positive concepts can play in the production of meaningful lives, fully functional families, and humanitarian societies that can actually promote health and healing. When expressed in this way, positivity becomes more than mere hedonistic pursuit of happiness—it becomes a universal aspiration. Rather than being accessible only to those in elite and privileged circumstances, positivity becomes something that can be sought after at all levels of society and across multiple sectors (Hart & Sasso, 2011). As Kristjánsson (2010) argued, positive ways of being, acting, and thinking can become a vehicle to a better society for all citizens.

The challenge that arises following a rapid growth in popularity of a concept such as positivity is that this natural process has the potential to become a tool for conservative cost-cutting political authorities. We have shown how other concepts, such as community rehabilitation, empowerment, and self-management (Kendall, Buys, & Larner, 2000; Kendall & Rogers, 2007), have become the focus of formal interventions aimed at reducing health care costs by enhancing outcomes and minimizing reliance on formal services. Although this action may initially be driven by the belief that such concepts are inherently valuable, formalizing the delivery of naturally occurring concepts in this way can actually prevent the translation of their value into reality. Well-meaning interventionists can inadvertently coopt these concepts, forcing them into artificial environments where they, ironically, no longer evolve naturally. As a result, positive concepts may fail to deliver the expected outcomes and may quickly drop out of favor.

Rather than focusing on the delivery of specific positive concepts through artificial interventions, it seems useful to instead focus on creating the general conditions under which positive qualities are likely to emerge. In 1996, we described such a framework for rehabilitation, which we called expansion rehabilitation (Newsome & Kendall, 1996). In this framework, we defined a model of rehabilitation based on the opportunity space that surrounds all individuals. The size and shape of this space was thought to be determined by the combination of circumstances, resources, and capabilities. Symbolically, this space represents the area within which an individual can easily move throughout their lifetime. An acquired disability undoubtedly results in displacement of this space and constriction of the opportunities available to the person and his or her family. Thus, the role of rehabilitation might be to simply expand the opportunity space around each individual, giving them more room to move if they choose to do so. Judgments about the location of the space that was occupied prior to or following the injury becomes irrelevant. Presumably, if opportunity can be expanded sufficiently, there may actually be an overlap with the preinjury space, but in other circumstances, entirely new spaces may be opened up for exploration. The decision about where to move within the new expanded space rests with the individual rather than with the professional. By defining rehabilitation in this way, the balance of power is shifted back to the individuals with the brain injury and they are given the freedom and support to choose the methods by which they take their opportunities to fruition.

Even if overarching positive frameworks such as expansion rehabilitation can be identified, implementation remains extremely challenging. Practice in this area lags well behind evidence. The tools and processes that dominate our system continue to manifest as negative rather than positive influences. In the brain injury area, this impact is complicated by the dominance of medicolegal processes and neuropsychological assessment that seeks to demonstrate deficits and document damages (Rowlands, 2001). However, in this book, we have shown that more positive processes can be deliberately engineered, thus allowing a much-needed focus on growth, flourishing and moral practices. We hope the chapters in this book help to chart a positive course for the future of brain injury rehabilitation.

References

Dunn, D. S., & Dougherty, S. B. (2005). Prospects for a positive psychology of rehabilitation. *Rehabilitation Psychology, 50*(3), 305–311.

Hart, K. E., & Sasso, T. (2011). Mapping the contours of contemporary positive psychology. *Canadian Psychology/Psychologie canadienne, 52*(2), 82–92.

Kendall, E., Buys, N.J., & Larner, J. (2000). Community-based service delivery in rehabilitation: The promise and the paradox. *Disability and Rehabilitation, 22*(10), 435–445.

Kendall, E., & Rogers, A. (2007). Extinguishing the social?: State sponsored self-care policy and the Chronic Disease Management Programme. *Disability & Society, 22*(2), 129–143.

Kristjánsson, K. (2010). Positive psychology, happiness, and virtue: The troublesome conceptual issues. *Review of General Psychology, 14*(4), 296–310.

McGrath, J. C. (2011). Posttraumatic growth and spirituality after brain injury. *Brain Impairment, 12*(2), 82–92.

Naidoo, P., van den Berg, H. S., & Hayes, G. (2006). Potential contributions to disability theorizing and research from positive psychology. *Disability and Rehabilitation, 28*(9), 595.

Newsome, R., & Kendall, E. (1996). Expansion rehabilitation: An empowering conceptual framework for rehabilitation following acquired disability. *Australian Journal of Rehabilitation Counseling, 2*(2), 71–85.

Rowlands, A. (2001). Ability or disability? Strengths-based practice in the area of traumatic brain injury. *Families in Society, 82*(3), 273.

Sunderland, N., Catalano, T., & Kendall, E. (2009). Missing discourses: Concepts of joy and happiness in disability. *Disability and Society, 24*(6), 703–714.

About the Editors and Contributors

EDITORS

Elizabeth Kendall, PhD, is a professor and research psychologist at Griffith University and the Centre for National Research on Disability and Rehabilitation (CONROD). She focuses on adjustment and self-management following acquired disability and chronic illness. She also examines innovative health service models that are responsive to diverse populations and the creation of healthy contexts (family, work, community, service systems) to accommodate disability, prevent injury, and/or promote health. Her research represents a holistic approach to the issues faced by people with disabilities and chronic conditions and can provide realistic, grounded responses to their needs. She has personal experience with acquired brain injury in her family and has advocated over the years for improved services.

Heidi Muenchberger, PhD, M.Psych. (Neuro), is an associate professor of environmental psychology at Griffith Health Institute, and has worked in the area of neurorehabilitation for the past 15 years. As a clinical neuropsychologist and research psychologist, she has primarily worked with people who have experienced a life-changing neurological disorder, and her research to date has concentrated on the impact of injury for individuals and their families. This work has informed her current research focus, which aims to investigate the broader environmental impact of place for people with catastrophic injury and illness encompassing social health and housing design.

John Wright has a degree in agricultural science with further training in disability studies, coaching, and education. He sustained an acquired brain injury as a child, although he and his family did not realize this for another 20 years when they sought help. With the support of his physiotherapist mother he regained full use of his paralyzed limbs. He has been a strong supporter for policies that protect people with brain injuries from inadequate services or stigma and harm. He has brought together his interests in multiple programs that combine outdoor or rural activities with therapeutic programs for people with disabilities including horse-riding to develop abilities and rural skills programs. He has developed programs for school children focused on farming and access to animals.

CONTRIBUTORS

Erica Anderson. Growing up in Southern Oregon, 21-year-old, Erica Anderson was exposed to storytelling through The Oregon Shakespeare Festival. It grew into imagination in the outdoors, which became the playground for childhood adventures. When she is not writing, she is horseback riding. This is a great way to confuse people. Many conversations go like this: "No. I am riding today, not writing." The equestrian world has always been a part of her identity. Erica would never have found writing without riding. It introduced her to the character, Velvet Brown, from *National Velvet*. Identity of character is a powerful thing, driving her into writing stories about her horse and her friends. Wherever life takes Erica, she will find time to own her writing ability and share the joy of storytelling along the journey.

Fiona Ashworth completed her doctorate in clinical psychology at the University of Oxford in September 2007. During her training, Fiona had a specialist placement at the Oxford Centre for Enablement, formally the Rivermead Rehabilitation Centre. She has worked as a clinical psychologist at the Oliver Zangwill Centre since qualifying in 2007. Fiona has a keen interest in the emotional and psychosocial impact of brain injury; she is particularly interested in the application of compassion focused therapy with people with acquired brain injury and has been researching and developing this approach at the Oliver Zangwill Centre. She has recently published an article outlining this approach and its application in brain injury. She is also studying for a postqualification masters in clinical neuropsychology at the University of Glasgow.

Martha E. Banks is a research neuropsychologist at ABackans DCP, Inc., in Akron, Ohio and a former professor of Black Studies at The College of Wooster. Prior to her retirement from the Brecksville Medical Center, she served as a clinical psychologist and computer trainer. Her primary research is on treatment of the consequences of intimate partner violence. She was the 2008–2009 president of the Society for the Psychology of Women. Martha is a fellow of the American Psychological Association. Martha's work as a psychologist has been recognized with an APA Presidential Citation and a President's Distinguished Achievement Award from the University of Rhode Island. A prolific author, she has published the 2003 book *Women with Visible and Invisible Disabilities: Multiple Intersections, Multiple Issues, Multiple Therapies*; the 2009 three-volume book set *Disabilities: Insights from across Fields and around the World*, and over 100 peer-reviewed encyclopedia entries, book chapters, and journal articles.

Glyn Blackett studied natural sciences at Cambridge University and then cognitive science at Manchester University. His involvement in therapy grew out of an interest in meditation. He first encountered biofeedback in the course of personal study of the mind–body relationship and was immediately struck by its therapeutic potential. Shortly after ward he began training in psychotherapy and hypnotherapy. His current interest in mindfulness-based psychotherapy was a natural development from his connection with meditation. His early experience in therapeutic practice was at a natural health clinic in Manchester. Later moving to York he established his current practice (York Biofeedback Centre) early in 2005. Glyn has also attended trainings in cognitive behavioral therapy (CBT), stress management, biofeedback, and neurofeedback.

Russell Bowen is a Guugu Yimidhirr man from Hope Vale. Russell worked with the Acquired Brain Injury Outreach Service (ABIOS, Queensland Health) on the Brain Injury Project in Cape York in 2006–2009. He attended the National Brain Injury Conference in Melbourne in 2008 with the project team, which further developed his interest in this area, and resulted in the Brain Injury Round Table in Cooktown in 2009, involving participants from four Cape York communities.

James S. Brady achieved a lifelong career goal when President Ronald Reagan appointed him assistant to the president and White House press secretary in January 1981. His service, however, was cut short on March 30, 1981, when a mentally deranged young man, John Hinckley, attempted to assassinate the president, and shot both President Reagan, Jim, and two law enforcement officers. Jim suffered a serious head wound that left him partially paralyzed for life. Since leaving the White House, Jim has spent countless hours lobbying with his wife Sarah, chair of the Brady Campaign to Prevent Gun Violence (formerly Handgun Control), for common sense gun laws.

Samantha Bursnall, BBehSc, Hons (psych), PhD, is a clinical psychologist working in a Child and Adolescent Mental Health Service (Generic CAMHS and Autism Team) within the Department of Child and Family at the Tavistock Centre, London. Samantha is also an Adjunct Principal Research Fellow at the Centre of National Research on Disability and Rehabilitation Medicine, Griffith University. She has a particular research and clinical interest in the impact of disability and illness on family members and has been involved with a number of published articles and book chapters on the subject both in Australia and the UK. Her research has focused on young carers, the impact of acquired brain injury on siblings, and parenting a child with autism and learning difficulties.

Anita Chauvin has worked with organizations and individuals within the health and human service sectors for 25 years. Her research has focused on developing, implementing, and evaluating population health promotion programs and clinical services across diverse health settings and populations (including HIV/AIDS, catastrophic trauma, social disadvantage, mental illness, and intellectual disability). She has a particular interest in change and growth after trauma, and her work has better informed the way we understand individual-level, as well as community-level, resilience and vulnerability. This important research has had direct impact on capacity building interventions across the world as has been particularly relevant in communities affected by natural and other disasters in more recent years. Anita has presented her work internationally.

Rudi Coetzer is a full-time clinician employed by BetsiCadwaladr University Health Board NHS Wales, United Kingdom. He is a consultant neuropsychologist and head of the North Wales Brain Injury Service. Rudi was appointed to this post during 1998 with the specific remit of developing a Pan-North Wales community-based neurorehabilitation service. Prior to this, he worked in a university teaching hospital setting. Rudi's clinical and academic interests are mainly within the field of brain injury rehabilitation, including psychotherapy approaches. He is an honorary senior lecturer in the School of Psychology at Bangor University.

Susan Gauld (Bachelor of Occupational Therapy, University of Queensland, 1981) is rehabilitation coordinator with the Acquired Brain Injury Outreach Service (ABIOS), Queensland Health. She has had many years' experience in community-based rehabilitation with adults with ABI and their families. Together with Sharon Smith she has initiated, developed, and implemented an integrated service model for Aboriginal and Torres Strait Islander adults with ABI, their families, and communities, which operates within a mainstream health service.

Lisa Guttentag Lederer, MA, is a graduate student in bioethics at the University of Pittsburgh. She has investigated head injury and the interaction between cognitive and social functioning from many angles, including from within cognitive psychology, communication science and disorders, and the history and philosophy of science. Her current research focuses on how disability impacts quality of life.

Maria Hennessy, PhD, M.Psych (Clinical), BA (Hons), MAPS, CCP, CCN, is a senior lecturer in the Department of Psychology at James Cook University, and has worked as a clinical psychologist and neuropsychologist for the past 18 years. As a clinical neuropsychologist, she has wide experience across the life span ranging from the assessment of childhood health disorders, traumatic brain injury, and dementia. Her recent role as a manager within Queensland Health led to the awarding of a Health Research Fellowship to investigate mental health outcomes following traumatic brain injury. Her current research continues this work, along with improving consumer participation rates in mental health services, and developing clinical measures to support outcome and recovery.

Melissa Kendall, PhD, is the research and development officer with the Acquired Brain Injury Outreach Service, a community rehabilitation program for people with acquired brain injury and the Transitional Rehabilitation Program, a community rehabilitation program for people with spinal cord injury. In 2009, she completed her doctor of philosophy investigating the value of friendships following traumatic injury. Her research interests include psychosocial adjustment following traumatic injury, discharge planning, community-based models of rehabilitation, and goal setting and attainment in rehabilitation. In addition to her own research, her current position involves building research capacity among health care practitioners working within spinal cord injury and brain injury rehabilitation in Queensland.

Areti Kennedy (Bachelor of Physiotherapy, Grad Dip Health Science). Areti has worked across the continuum in brain injury rehabilitation, from the acute setting, through hospital rehabilitation and into the community for the past 18 years. From 1997–2005, she was a rehabilitation coordinator at the Acquired Brain Injury Outreach Service (ABIOS), a tertiary rehabilitation service for adults with brain injury their families and service providers across Queensland. From 2005–2008, she was the Project Officer, Skills To Enable People and Communities (STEPS) Project at ABIOS, which aimed to establish a model by which sustainable, self-managed networks of support for people with acquired brain injury and their families in local communities around Queensland could be established. She was the recipient of a Health and Community Services Workforce Council award for Workforce Innovation in 2011 and a finalist in the Queensland Health Healthcare Improvement awards in 2011.

Pim Kuipers, PhD, is an associate professor and principal research fellow with the Centre for Functioning and Health Research (Queensland Health) and the Population and Social Health Research Program, Griffith Health Institute (Griffith University). His research interests include health service delivery, rural and remote services, community-based rehabilitation, and services to people with brain injuries and people with spinal cord injuries.

Paul Leung, PhD, is currently professor, Department of Rehabilitation, Social Work and Addictions, University of North Texas. Paul previously held academic/administrative appointments at Deakin University (Melbourne, Australia), the University of Illinois (Urbana), the University of North Carolina at Chapel Hill and the University of Arizona. He has served as past president of Division 22 (Rehabilitation Psychology) of the American Psychological Association, the National Council on Rehabilitation Education, and the National Association of Multicultural Rehabilitation Concerns. A former editor of the *Journal of Rehabilitation*, his research interests have centered on persons with disabilities from diverse ethnic/racial groups and rehabilitation. He has been honored with the Sylvia Walker National Multicultural Award from the National Rehabilitation Association, the Lifetime Achievement Award from Division 22 of the American Psychological Association, the Vergie-Winston Smith Lifetime Achievement Award from the National Association of Multicultural Rehabilitation Concerns, and the Distinguished Career in Rehabilitation Education Award from the National Council on Rehabilitation Education.

Michelle McIntyre is a senior research assistant at the Population and Social Health Research Program, Griffith Health Institute, Griffith University. Michelle has a background in education and learning theory. Her doctoral studies focus on the family experience of traumatic brain injury, with a specific interest in family resources and resilience over time. Other research interests include health systems, responses to health care complexity, and health promotion.

Kenneth I. Pakenham, PhD, is an associate professor in clinical and health psychology in the School of Psychology at The University of Queensland, Australia. He has published over 100 refereed journal articles on disability, illness, and caregiving. In particular, he and colleagues have pioneered measurement and theory development research in young caregiving.

Hayley Danielle Quinn, BPsych (Hons) is a PhD (clinical psychology) candidate at Griffith University, Brisbane, Australia. Her research is focused on the experience of home for young people with disabilities living in long term residential care. She completed her bachelor of psychology (Honours) in 2007 with research evaluating interventions to improve metacognitive skills during an everyday activity following traumatic brain injury. Hayley is a clinical psychologist registrar and works in private practice. She also works at a private psychiatric hospital where she facilitates a group day program that provides focused treatment for people experiencing significant distress and dysfunction associated with trauma. She is an associate member of the Australian Psychological Society and a committee member for the Australian Association of Cognitive Behavioral Therapy.

Sharon Smith is a Rehabilitation Coordinator (Social Worker) with the Acquired Brain Injury Outreach Service (ABIOS), a community rehabilitation service for adults with acquired brain injury. Sharon was lead investigator (with her colleague, Susan Gauld) on the three-year research project working with remote Indigenous communities (2006–09) to develop the most suitable and culturally appropriate community-based service model for Aboriginal and Torres Strait Islander adults with acquired brain injury and their families. With colleagues, she has developed and implemented a training program for health workers on brain injury.

Susan Wenberg, PhD, owns a private practice in Tucson Arizona offering health care services for patients of all ages. She has been a board member, speaker chair, and education committee cochair of NORA (Neuro-Optometric Rehabilitation Association, International, Inc.), an association of clinicians and educators concerned with meeting the needs of individuals with traumatic brain injuries. Susan is a Professional Advisory Board Member of Polio Epic, a Tucson-based support group for those with Post Polio Syndrome. In 1981, on the last day of a 90-day bicycle tour across the United States, she sustained multiple injuries including a mild traumatic brain injury. She was introduced to chiropractic four years postinjury, while studying biomechanics. Susan holds a doctor of chiropractic degree from Los Angeles College of Chiropractic, a master's degree from UCLA, and a BA from Linfield College in Oregon. She continues to bicycle tour; she has toured self-contained across the United States, Iceland, the Czech Republic, and Estonia.

Barbara A. Wilson is a clinical neuropsychologist who has worked in brain injury rehabilitation for 35 years. She has won many awards for her work including an OBE for services to medical rehabilitation in 1998 and two lifetime achievement awards, one from the British Psychological Society and one from the International Neuropsychological Society. In 2011 she received the Ramon Y. Cahal award from the International Neuropsychiatric Association. She has published 18 books, over 270 journal articles and chapters, and 8 neuropsychological tests. She is editor of the journal *Neuropsychological Rehabilitation*, which she founded in 1991 and in 1996 she founded the Oliver Zangwill Centre for Neuropsychological Rehabilitation. A rehabilitation center in Quito, Ecuador is named after her. She is currently president of the Encephalitis Society, vice president of the Academy for Multidisciplinary Neurotrauma, and on the management committee of The World Federation of Neuro Rehabilitation. The Division of Neuropsychology has named a prize after her, the Barbara A. Wilson prize for distinguished contributions to neuropsychology. She is a fellow of the British Psychological Society, the Academy of Medical Sciences, and the Academy of Social Sciences.

Jill Winegardner is a clinical neuropsychologist with 30 years of experience in brain injury assessment and rehabilitation. She has worked in a range of settings including acute inpatient, acute and postacute rehabilitation, residential rehabilitation, and outpatient care. She founded and directed the Cleveland Metro Brain Injury Rehabilitation Program, where she worked for five years before moving to Nicaragua for several years to help establish the field of neuropsychology in that country. She is currently lead clinical psychologist at the Oliver Zangwill Centre for Neuropsychological Rehabilitation in Ely, UK. Her clinical and research interests include neuropsychological assessment and programmer design and evaluation.

BAKER COLLEGE LIBRARY

3 3504 00585 6655

RC 387.5 .H43 2013

Health and healing after
traumatic brain injury

DATE DUE

GAYLORD   #3522PI   Printed in USA

Property of
Baker College
of Allen Park